HEALTH & WELLNESS SERIES

DIABETES ESSENTIALS

EVERYDAY BASICS

Tips & Recipes to Manage Type 2 Diabetes

KAREN GRAHAM, RD, CDE
Registered Dietitian &
Certified Diabetes Educator

MANSUR SHOMALI, MD, CM
Endocrinologist & Diabetes Expert

....

JANICE MADILL, BSW, BSc
Senior Editor

Robert
ROSE

Diabetes Essentials: Tips & Recipes to Manage Type 2 Diabetes

Disclaimer

The suggestions and information contained in this publication are based on a thorough assessment of the latest research and information. Reasonable steps have been taken to ensure the accuracy of the information presented. However, we cannot ensure the safety or efficacy of any product or service described in this publication. Individuals are advised to consult a physician or other appropriate health care professional before undertaking any diet, exercise, activity or treatment program or taking any herb or medication referred to in this publication. Professionals must use and apply their own professional judgment, experience, and training and should not rely solely on the information contained in this publication before prescribing any diet, exercise, treatment or medication. While we thank the professional expertise of the reviewers of this publication, neither they nor the authors or publisher assumes any responsibility or liability for personal or other injury, loss or damage that may result from the suggestions or information in this publication.

The recipes in this book have been carefully tested by our kitchen and our tasters. To the best of our knowledge, they are safe and nutritious for ordinary use and users. For those people with food or other allergies, or who have special food requirements or health issues, please read the suggested contents of each recipe carefully and determine whether or not they may create a problem for you. All recipes are used at the risk of the consumer. For those with special needs, allergies, requirements or health problems, in the event of any doubt, please contact your medical adviser prior to the use of any recipe.

This book is not intended as a substitute for professional medical care. Only your doctor can diagnose and treat a medical problem.

Use of brand names is for educational purposes only and does not imply endorsement.

Library and Archives Canada Cataloguing in Publication

Title: Diabetes essentials : tips & recipes to manage type 2 diabetes / Karen Graham, RD, CDE, Registered Dietitian & Certified Diabetes Educator, Mansur Shomali, MD, CM, endocrinologist and diabetes expert ; Janice Madill, BSW, BSc, senior editor.
Names: Graham, Karen, author. | Shomali, Mansur, author. | Madill, Janice, 1956- editor.
Description: Series statement: Health & wellness series | Includes index.
Identifiers: Canadiana 20190207833 | ISBN 9780778806318 (softcover)
Subjects: LCSH: Diabetes—Popular works.
Classification: LCC RC660.4 .G73 2020 | DDC 616.4/62—dc23

Senior Editor: Janice Madill, Easy English
Robert Rose Proof Editor and Proofreader: Sue MacLeod
Robert Rose Recipe Editor: Sue Sumeraj
Early Process Editor: Joanne Seiff
Reviewers: Margaret Graham; Dr. Carl Durand, OD, for the eye section.
Design and Production: Alicia McCarthy & Joseph Gisini/PageWave Graphics Inc.
Cover Design: Kevin Cockburn/PageWave Graphics Inc.
Nutrient Analysis: Karen Graham, RD, CDE, based on American and Canadian nutrient files, and food labels as applicable.
Recipe Contributors: Carl Durand, Carl's Red Cabbage Slaw (p 83); Urbania Buckner, Bonnie's Potato Salad (p 86).

Image Credits

Photos and illustrations are from Getty Images except as noted below. Any person depicted in Getty Images content is a model.
p 6: Dr. Shomali with patient © April Arnold; p 12 (tablets), p 21 (foot screen) & p 182 (weights): © Brian Gould; p 31 (kitchen) & p 43 (dining) © Andrew Lipsett; p 44: Hand illustration chart © Durand & Graham Ltd. / Graphic artwork © Sandi Storen; p 66 (Karen Graham in the kitchen) & back cover (Karen Graham) © David McIlvride / Jenny McKinney, Makeup artist; Back cover (Dr. Shomali) © Juliette Bogus.

The publisher gratefully acknowledges the financial support of our publishing program by the Government of Canada through the Canada Book Fund.

Canadä

Published by Robert Rose Inc.
120 Eglinton Avenue East, Suite 800, Toronto, Ontario, Canada M4P 1E2
Tel: (416) 322-6552 Fax: (416) 322-6936
www.robertrose.ca

Printed and bound in South Korea

2 3 4 5 6 7 8 9 FC 28 27 26 25 24 23 22 21 20

UP-TO-DATE INFORMATION ABOUT DIABETES!

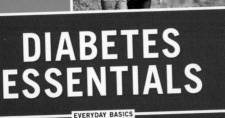
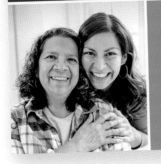
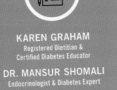

HEALTH & WELLNESS SERIES

STARTER BOOK

DIABETES ESSENTIALS

EVERYDAY BASICS

Tips & Recipes to Manage Type 2 Diabetes

KAREN GRAHAM
Registered Dietitian &
Certified Diabetes Educator

DR. MANSUR SHOMALI
Endocrinologist & Diabetes Expert

ABOUT DIABETES ESSENTIALS

This book is organized into short and easy *top-ten lists*. Start with "Diabetes First Ten Days" on pages 12–13. These are easy things to do right away.

After the first ten days, take a deep breath. You've begun to make some changes. You don't have to change everything at once. When you are ready, read some of the other top-ten diabetes topics. Along the way you can do some of the quizzes. Make and enjoy some of the easy and delicious recipes for yourself and your family. Read the table of contents and choose the topics that are most important to you.

Keep in regular contact with your doctor and health care providers. Follow their medical advice about what is right for you.

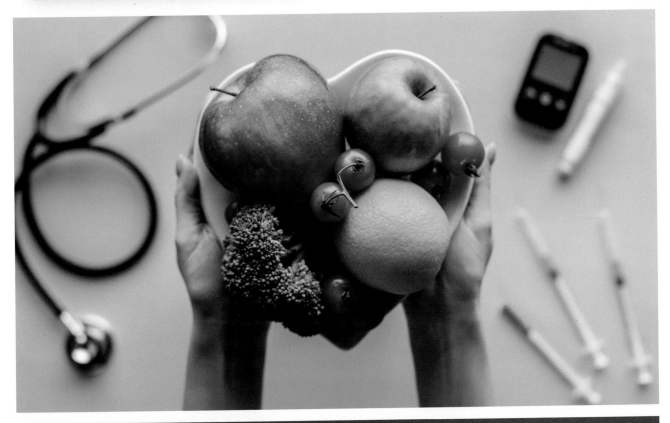

FOR OTHER BOOKS IN OUR HEALTH & WELLNESS SERIES, SEE PAGE 192.

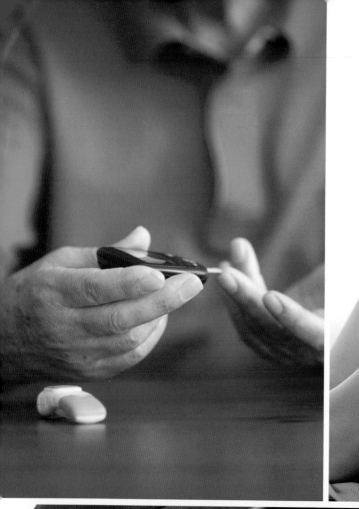
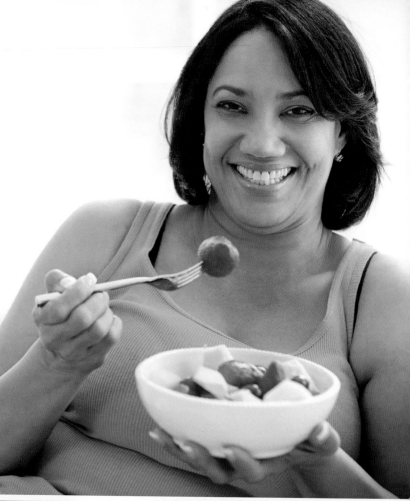
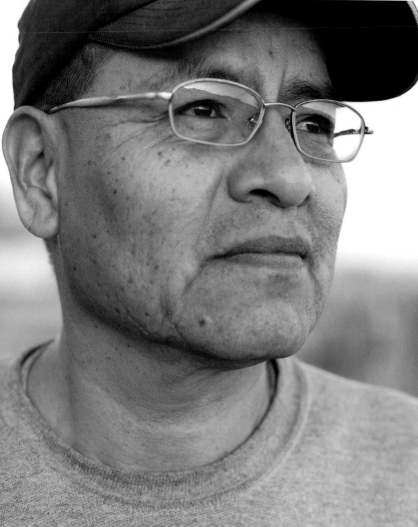
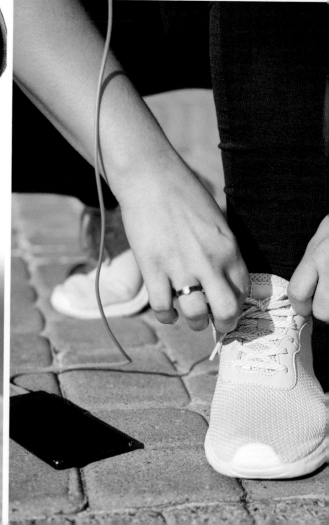

Contents

Thank You to:

1 **Janice Madill, Senior Editor.** With our ideas, stories and medical knowledge of diabetes, the authors have written too many pages to count. Janice Madill of Easy English has helped write this book, making it easy-to-read, well organized and appealing. As well as being an outstanding editor, Janice is a compassionate social worker. She understands what needs to be said.

2 **Patients and clients.** During our combined 50 years of experience as a diabetes educator and an expert physician, we have counseled thousands of people with diabetes. They have shared with us their practical experiences of living with diabetes. Thanks to them, we can now share this knowledge with you.

3 **Bob Dees and Robert Rose Inc.** For nearly 30 years, Robert Rose has been a wellness leader through the publication of cookbooks and healthy lifestyle books. Bob Dees, President of Robert Rose, is highly dedicated to publishing, and is involved in the layout and content of every book. We would like to thank Bob and his production, sales and marketing staff: Kelly Glover and Megan Brush. Thanks also to Sue MacLeod, proof editor, and Gillian Watts, indexer.

4 **PageWave Graphics.** PageWave has been creatively designing books for more than 20 years. Under the guidance of Joseph Gisini, designer Alicia McCarthy has helped select meaningful photographs. Alicia has designed beautiful color schemes and layouts for this stunning book.

Dr. Shomali says "Every day, we learn from patients about their efforts to manage their diabetes."

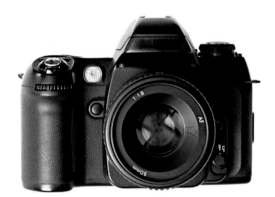

5 **The photographers.** Beautiful photographs help convey to you, the reader, the complexities of diabetes. We are grateful for these images, and the visual learning we can provide for you.

6 **Diabetes associations.** Organizations such as the American Diabetes Association and Diabetes Canada develop diabetes clinical practice guidelines, which help guide the work of diabetes health care professionals. These organizations also help fund advanced diabetes research.

7 **Diabetes educators.** These are the professionals who help you learn about diabetes, who help you manage your personal struggles with diabetes and who listen to your worries. They take the time to coach you and give you their best advice with problems as they arise. Thank you diabetes educators for your commitment in the fight against diabetes.

8 **Family and friends.** Who would we be without them? They are the special people who surround us; they know us, they accept us and they care about us.

9 **Home cooking.** Home-cooked meals are healthier than any fast food or prepared frozen food. The delicious recipes in this book have been home-tested by Karen Graham and her team. Gather your friends and family together and enjoy making these meals.

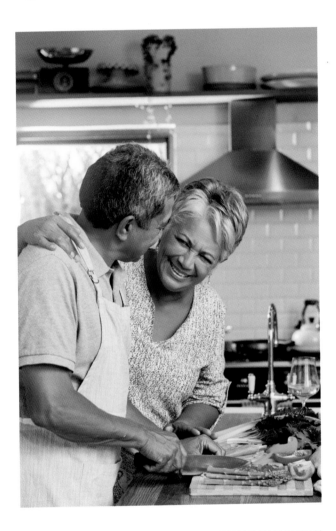

10 **A special thank you to Rick Durand.** Karen's husband, Rick Durand, is an innovative and creative thinker, which has been exemplified during his career as a plant breeder. Over the past five years, Rick's interest in this book brought out his many novel ideas that kept this book moving in exciting directions.

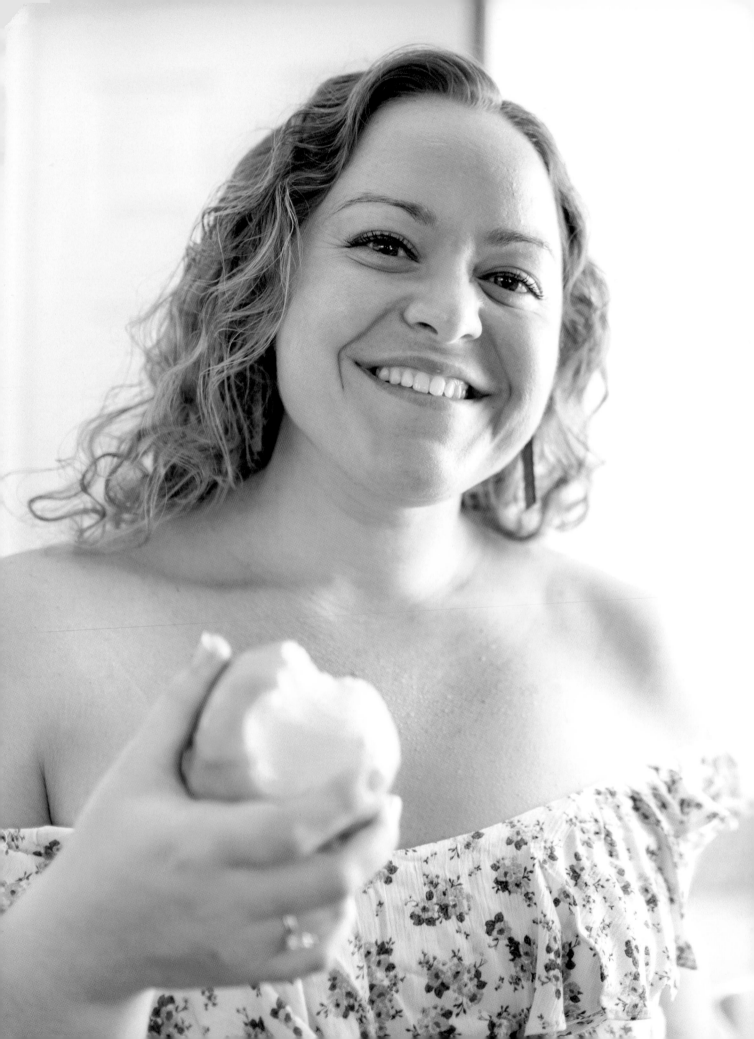

Get Started

Prediabetes

1 **Prediabetes is a condition where your blood sugar (blood glucose) is higher than normal.** An A1C test of 5.7 to 6.4% in the USA, or 6 to 6.4% in Canada, is considered prediabetes. This lab test measures the amount of sugar in your blood over the past three months.

2 **You will not have any diabetes symptoms.** For example, you will not feel extra thirst or hunger or have slow-healing sores. You can have prediabetes for many years without knowing, before it progresses to type 2 diabetes.

3 **How do you know if you have prediabetes?** Only with an A1C test. Get tested if you're over 45, or sooner if you're overweight or have a family history.

4 **Prediabetes can cause early damage to your heart.** Statistics show that people with prediabetes have more heart attacks than people who don't have prediabetes.

5 **Take prediabetes seriously.** If changes are made at the prediabetes stage, there is a very good chance that type 2 diabetes can be prevented.

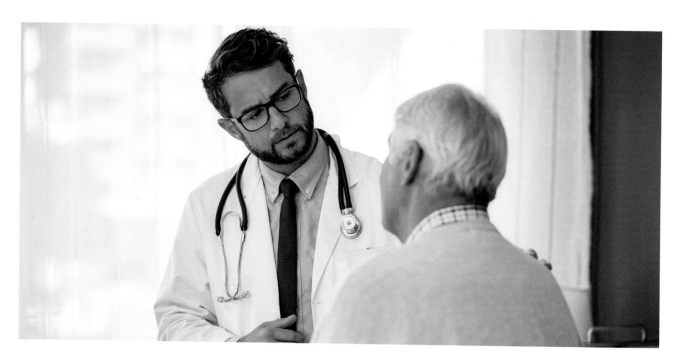

6 **Make one diet change right away.**
For example, cut back or cut out sweet drinks like regular soft drinks, juices, sweetened coffees and teas, sports and energy drinks, and sweetened smoothies and milkshakes. You will lose a few pounds, which will help bring down your blood sugar.

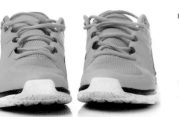

7 **Become more active right away.** Don't delay. Start with a short 15-minute walk every day.

8 **Your doctor may prescribe a diabetes medication for you.** Don't be surprised — metformin is often prescribed for prediabetes, to bring your blood sugar back to normal. But lifestyle changes are important too. Studies have shown that they may be even more effective than medications.

9 **Blood pressure and cholesterol medication may also be helpful.** These may be prescribed at this time if you are not already taking them. They can help protect your heart and your kidneys.

10 **Children can also get prediabetes.** Consider this news as a chance to prevent type 2 diabetes in your children. See a dietitian and learn about healthy eating and exercise for your family.

When you teach your child to eat healthy foods and be active every day, this will lead to better choices as an adult. This means less chance of getting diabetes.

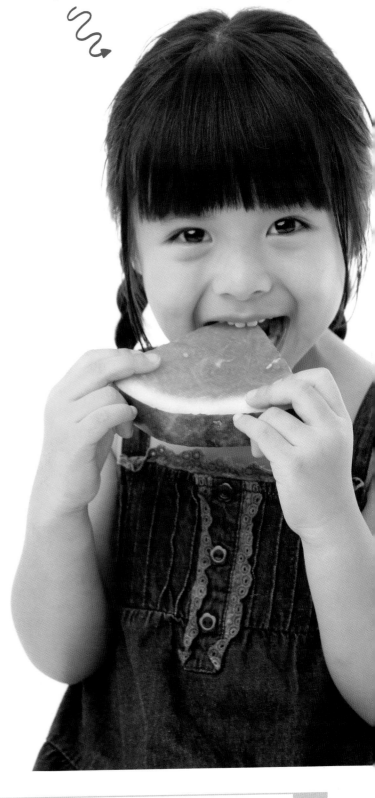

Diabetes First Ten Days

DAY 1 Take the pills or insulin your doctor has prescribed. Use a pill organizer to sort your pills for the week. Buy a journal today, special or practical, because you are going to want to make notes as time goes on.

DAY 2 This is a good day to find out what your blood sugar number is. Ask a pharmacist or nurse to check it. Or, try checking it yourself if you know how, and if you feel ready to start doing that.

DAY 3 Start your day today with breakfast. Note in your journal when you eat your daily meals and snacks. It is important to eat at the same time every day to help keep your blood sugar balanced.

DAY 4 Fill a large glass with water. While you are drinking your water, spend time today to write down your favorite high-sugar foods and drinks. This includes any soft drinks, iced teas, energy drinks, sweetened coffees and any cookies, donuts, ice creams and pastries.

DAY 5 Today, choose from your list of favorites, which foods and drinks you will start to eat and drink less of. Pills and insulin alone cannot control your diabetes; you have to cut back on sugary foods and drinks. Be proud of yourself — this is a good start for a new routine and a healthier you.

DAY 6 Now that you've cut back on sugary foods, you may feel a bit dizzy. It's okay; it's a positive sign that your blood sugar is coming down. Rest and have a drink of water and the dizzy feeling will pass. However, if you've started on insulin, treat this as a low blood sugar episode instead. Take 3 to 5 glucose tablets (15 grams in total) or a tablespoon of sugar. See page 28 for a more complete list.

To treat a low blood sugar episode, you need fast-acting carbohydrates — in other words, sugars that absorb quickly into your bloodstream. Glucose tablets work the fastest since glucose is the same type of sugar that is already in your blood. Fifteen grams of glucose equals 15 grams of carbohydrate.

DAY 7 Check your feet today.
Look them all over for any small marks or sores. It is important to keep your feet clean. Gently rub some hand cream on any dry areas, especially on your heels. Wear shoes that fit properly.

DAY 8 Now that your feet are ready, today is a great day to go for a walk.
Start with a short stroll and enjoy the outdoors, whatever the season. Go easy; too much exercise too soon when your sugars are high can actually increase your blood sugar. Congratulations, you're through the first week!

DAY 9 Take time today to write down all the changes you've made and check back with your health care team.
More than a week has passed, so it's a good time to go back to them with questions. Ask them to check your blood sugar, to see if your level has changed. Remember that not all treatments start to work right away.

DAY 10 Treat day!
All the changes you've made to eat and drink differently as a person with diabetes are not easy. Learn how to take moments to sit still, relax with no interruptions and breathe. This is part of your balance.

Enjoy a 50 gram ($1\frac{1}{2}$ oz) chocolate bar or similar-size treat.

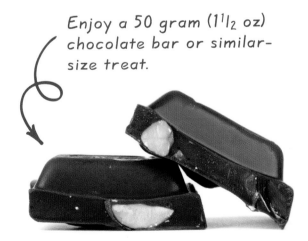

Appointments

1 Your questions. In the beginning you will have many questions. Write them down. For all appointments with your doctor and other health care providers bring your list of questions with you.

2 Doctor, Physician Assistant or Nurse Practitioner. Your health care provider will tell you about your diagnosis, prescribe and adjust medications and tell you what you need to do right away. They may refer you to a diabetes education center.

3 Diabetes Nurse Educator. This is a registered nurse who specializes in diabetes, offering group classes or individual assessment and education. You will get your questions answered about your lab results, your medications, or how you can prevent diabetes-related complications. Often, these nurse educators work at diabetes education centers along with dietitians.

4 Registered Dietitian. A dietitian will help you make healthy changes to your diet and improve your blood sugar. Dietitians can answer any food or diet questions.

5 Pharmacist. Diabetes treatment involves several medications, such as insulin and diabetes and blood pressure pills. It's important to use the same pharmacy for all your drugs so they will have a complete list.

6 Optometrist or Ophthalmologist. Set an appointment to see an eye doctor as soon as you find out you have diabetes. Ask for a Diabetes Eye Exam. The doctor will dilate your eyes with eye drops to check the blood vessels at the back of your eye. You will need someone to drive you home after this appointment.

7 Dentist. Gum infections are more likely when you have diabetes. See your dentist at least once a year.

8 Counselor. The mental stress of having diabetes can be overwhelming. Many workplaces provide free access to mental health counseling for employees. Or ask your doctor for a referral to a professional counselor. Talking with a trained professional will help you understand and manage your emotions as you make changes.

9 Family or friends. These are the people you trust and who support you over time. They can go with you to appointments and listen to what is being said in case you forget.

10 Diabetes books. If you need some more information, ask your health care provider to recommend a website or book that has accurate information. You can refer to them any time and as often as you need.

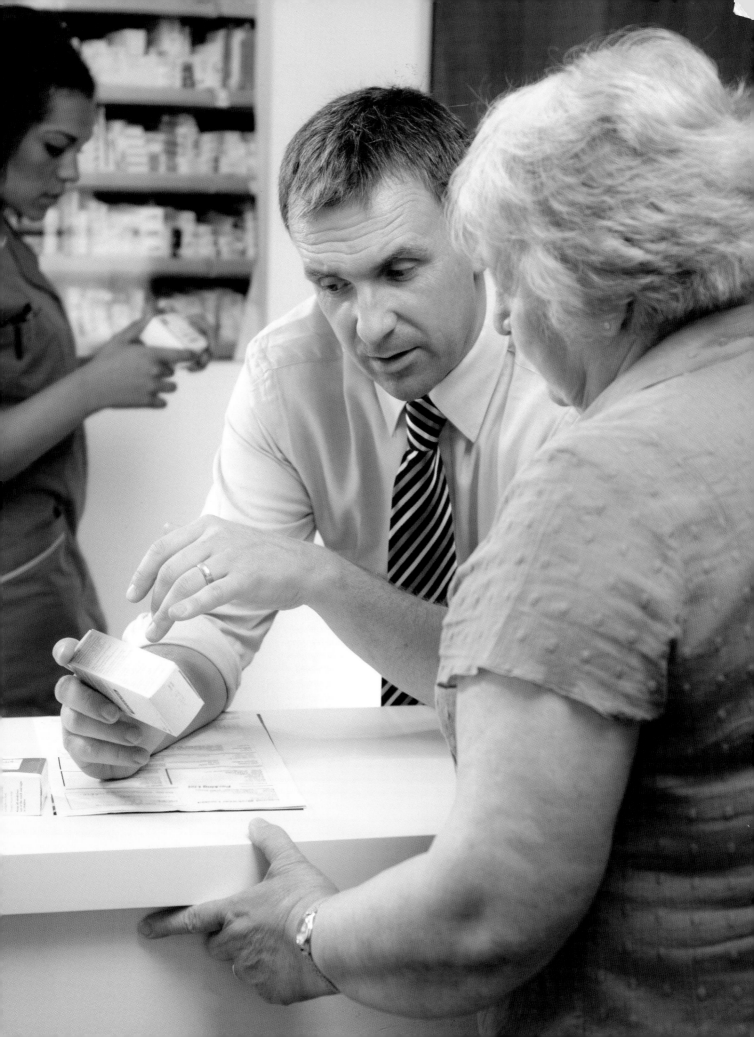

Answers to Your First Diabetes Questions

1 **What does prediabetes mean?** It means your blood sugar is higher than normal but not high enough to be type 2 diabetes. This is the time to make changes to your habits because you can significantly delay or prevent the start of diabetes.

2 **What is type 2 diabetes?** This is when there is too much sugar in your blood. Your body has changed and there is not enough insulin, or your insulin can no longer efficiently remove sugar from your blood. Type 2 diabetes is a progressive disease that needs to be treated to prevent or reduce harmful health complications over time.

3 **Do I really have diabetes?** Since you may not have obvious symptoms, a blood test will confirm if you have diabetes. Results from one of three common lab tests are a diagnosis of type 2 diabetes:

- a fasting blood sugar of 125 mg/dL USA (7 mmol/L CAN) or more, taken before you eat in the morning
- A1C of 6.5% or more
- a random blood sugar of 200 mg/dL USA (11.1 mmol/L CAN) or more, taken any time of the day.

Canada and America use different blood sugar measures. The United States uses standard mg/dL. Canada uses metric mmol/L. To convert mg/dL to mmol/L divide by 18. To convert mmol/L to mg/dL multiply by 18.

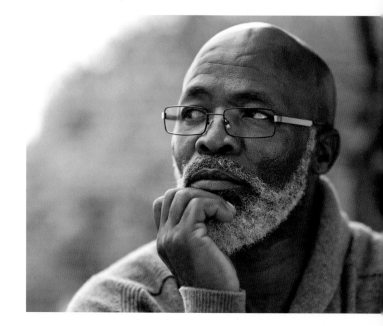

4 **Why did I get diabetes?** The causes of type 2 diabetes are complicated and not fully understood. They include our family genes, our childhood upbringing, our adult lifestyle, and even the community we live in. As you age or put on weight, or become less physically active, your body changes. Over time your body is not able to cope with extra sugar in your blood and you get diabetes.

5 **How bad is my diabetes?** Blood sugars can be high when you are first diagnosed but can improve once you cut out the sugary drinks and foods and start walking. When you start on medications, it takes weeks or longer for them to work. So, take your A1C test every three months and your doctor will monitor your progress.

6 Will I need to take insulin? Diabetes pills are usually the first medication started. Over time you may need more medication, which may include insulin. Some people never need insulin.

7 Will I have to prick my finger for blood every day? Knowing your blood sugar number can help you understand how well your medications, food choices and exercise are working. Most people don't need to check their blood sugar daily. If you are on insulin, you may need more frequent checking; ask about new continuous glucose monitors that mean fewer finger pricks.

8 What can I eat? You can continue to eat what you have always eaten, but you will have to eat less. High fat and high sugar foods cannot be daily foods. Enjoy them but a lot less often.

9 How do I get rid of diabetes? Type 2 diabetes cannot be cured, but it can be managed. Take your medications, change how much you eat and what you eat, become more physically active and you can help your body become healthier.

10 What if I can't make the changes? It is normal to feel this way. You will surprise yourself how one small change can make you feel better. Then it will feel easier to make another small change.

Diabetes Medical Terms

1 **Target blood sugar.** Blood sugar is also called blood glucose. For most people with diabetes, the recommended blood sugar level before a meal is about 80–130 mg/dL USA (4–7 mmol/L CAN). After a meal, blood sugar can go up to 180 mg/dL (10 mmol/L) but should quickly come back down.

2 **A1C.** The A-one-C is a single diabetes test taken once every three months (four times a year). This test is an average of the highs and lows of sugar in your blood over three months. Generally, you want your A1C to be 7% or lower.

3 **Hyperglycemia.** Hyper means high; glycemia means blood sugar. This is when blood sugar goes above 180 mg/dL USA (10 mmol/L CAN).

4 **Hypoglycemia.** Hypo means low; glycemia means blood sugar. This is when blood sugar level is under 70 mg/dL USA (4.0 mmol/L CAN). A person will feel dizzy and weak and will need to eat or drink sugar in some form.

5 **Insulin resistance.** Insulin is made in the pancreas. After you eat, insulin is released into your bloodstream to move sugar into the muscle cells and liver. Extra fat blocks insulin from moving sugar into these cells, so the sugar stays in the bloodstream. That is insulin resistance.

6 **Leaky liver.** The liver is not working properly. The liver naturally stores sugar, so if a meal is missed, it releases sugar into the bloodstream for a boost of energy. For a person with type 2 diabetes, the liver leaks sugar when it's not needed. This causes high blood sugar in the morning or other times of the day when not expected.

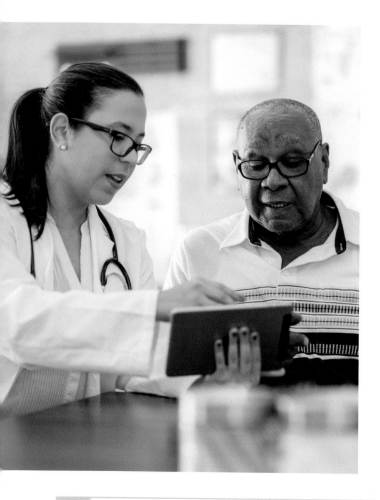

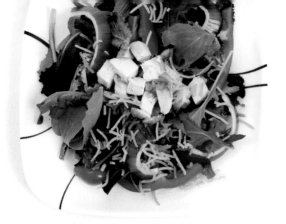

9 **Type 2 diabetes.** It is the most common type of diabetes in adults and tends to run in families. People with type 2 diabetes have high blood sugar, often with insulin resistance and a leaky liver. Although less common, it can occur in children or teenagers.

7 **Prediabetes.** Prediabetes means blood sugar levels are starting to rise above normal but not enough to be diagnosed as type 2 diabetes. When people with prediabetes start on a healthy path, such as eating better and exercising, they can prevent or delay type 2 diabetes.

10 **Gestational diabetes.** This is a short-term type of diabetes during pregnancy. It's more likely for women who have an excess weight gain and a family history of type 2 diabetes. These women and their babies are at risk of developing type 2 diabetes later. This risk is lessened with healthy eating and exercise.

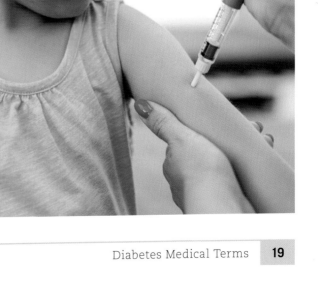

8 **Type 1 diabetes.** Type 1 diabetes is the most common type of diabetes in children and teenagers. This is a disease of the pancreas, which stops making insulin. Those with type 1 diabetes need insulin every day. Adults and older individuals can sometimes develop type 1 diabetes, which can confuse patients and health care professionals.

Lab Tests

1 **A1C ("A-one-C").** This test is taken every three months and measures how much sugar has built up in your blood during this time. You do not have to fast (skip eating) for this test, so it can be taken at any time of the day. If your A1C is high, your blood sugar is high. When several of your A1C tests are closer to normal blood sugar levels, they 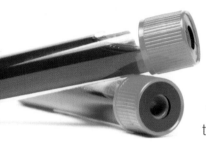 show you have made some positive and successful long-term changes. Then, you may only need to take an A1C test twice a year.

2 **Cholesterol.** Tests for cholesterol are part of the standard series of blood tests taken once a year. There are two types of cholesterol — good cholesterol (called HDL) and bad cholesterol (called LDL). It is the bad cholesterol that narrows your blood vessels. Narrow blood vessels will increase your blood pressure, which can increase your risk for diabetes complications.

3 **Blood pressure.** This is a standard test at all doctor's appointments. High blood pressure means your heart is working hard to pump the blood around in your body. High blood pressure can lead to heart failure, heart attacks and strokes. It can damage the blood vessels in your eyes and can worsen the function of your kidneys. Some people may benefit from checking their blood pressure at home with an automated meter.

4 **Kidney tests — ACR and eGFR.** These tests are taken at diagnosis and then once a year to measure how well your kidneys work. They help to alert the doctor of potential problems. ACR (Albumin Creatinine Ratio) measures protein leaking out of your kidneys into your urine. eGFR (estimated Glomerular Filtration Rate) measures the rate of fluid flowing through your kidney filters.

5 **Dilated eye exam.** Have an eye exam soon after your diagnosis of diabetes. The eye doctor puts drops in your eyes so the pupils dilate (expand). This allows a clear look to the back of your eyes. The eye doctor can see the tiny blood vessels and see any changes related to diabetes.

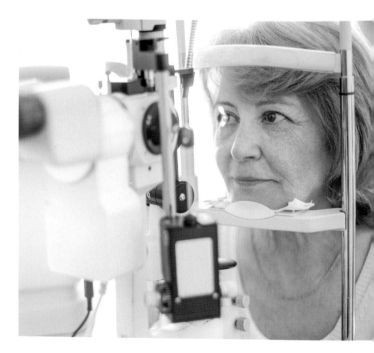

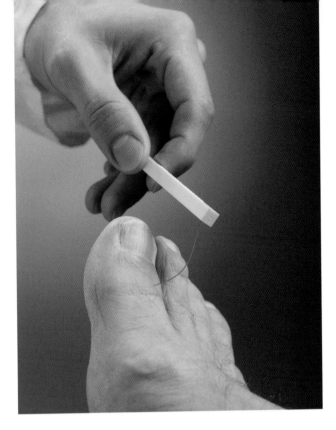

8 **Electrocardiogram at rest (ECG).** This test measures the electrical activity of your heart. An ECG can reveal an undiagnosed problem such as enlarged heart, which may be caused by high blood pressure. If you have had diabetes for at least 15 years and you are over 40 or have ever had a heart attack or other heart problem, this is an important test for you.

9 **Body weight.** Your weight may be checked at doctor's appointments to monitor weight losses or gains. One main goal for people with diabetes is to prevent weight gain. Dietitians and diabetes educators know that people can gain 10 pounds (4 to 5 kg) of extra weight over a year and not realize it.

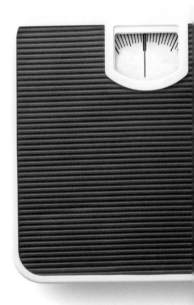

6 **Foot screen.** A foot screen is a pain-free, three-part test by a nurse or doctor. First is a simple test called a monofilament test. The bottom and top of each foot is touched with a small instrument. This tells how much nerve sensation you have. Second, the blood flow (pulse) to your feet and ankles will be checked. Third, your feet will be checked for sores or calluses or other physical changes.

10 **Depression test.** Depression is more common when you have diabetes. If you think you might be depressed, talk to your doctor about how you feel. After doing an assessment, the doctor may recommend exercise, counseling, medication or some other treatment.

7 **Dental exam.** When your blood sugar is high you have more sugar in your saliva. Bacteria grow on this extra sugar in your mouth. A dentist will clean and fix your teeth and will look for signs of bacterial infection (gum disease). If you have a bacterial infection, your body will naturally try to fight the infection, which produces stress hormones, which cause your blood sugar to go even higher. This is why taking care of your teeth and gums is so important.

Diabetes Medications

Health professionals study and rate diabetes drugs based on four main questions:

1. **A1C Benefit:** Does it lower blood sugar, based on A1C?

2. **Hypoglycemia/Low Blood Sugar:** Does it cause low blood sugar episodes?

3. **Initial weight change:** Does it influence weight in one of the following four ways? Weight loss (3½–7 lbs/1.6–3.0 kg), more weight loss (7–9 lbs/3–4 kg), weight gain (3–5½ lbs/1.5–2.5 kg) or more weight gain (5½–11 lbs/2.5–5kg)

4. **Benefit for your heart, blood vessels (vascular) or kidneys:** Does it reduce your chance of a heart attack or stroke, heart failure or kidney damage?

Your prescription will depend on your blood sugar level, weight, age and the health of your heart and kidneys. Your doctor will also look at side effects, cost and convenience of a drug for you. Diabetes drugs can slow the disease's progression and help you live a healthy life.

1 Metformin. Metformin (brand name Glucophage) helps prevent sugar leaking out of your liver. You will need to take a pill several times a day. Glumetza is a type of metformin that you can take just once a day.

A1C BENEFIT: Very Good. **HYPOGLYCEMIA:** Rare. **WEIGHT:** No weight change.

2 Insulin Secretagogues. These drugs help your pancreas make more insulin. These drug names end in "ide" such as gliclazide (Diamicron), glyburide (Diabeta), glimepiride (Amaryl), repaglinide (Prandin) and nateglinide (Starlix). They can cause weight gain and low blood sugar episodes.

A1C BENEFIT: Good. **HYPOGLYCEMIA:** Yes. **WEIGHT:** Weight gain.

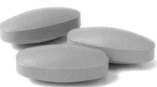

3 DPP-4 Inhibitors. These pills increase incretin hormones made in your intestines so your body makes more insulin when your blood sugar is high. These drug names end in "liptin" such as sitagliptin (Januvia), saxagliptin (Onglyza), linagliptin (Tragenta) and alogliptin (Nesina). These drugs are one pill a day.

A1C BENEFIT: Fair. **HYPOGLYCEMIA:** Rare. **WEIGHT:** No weight change.

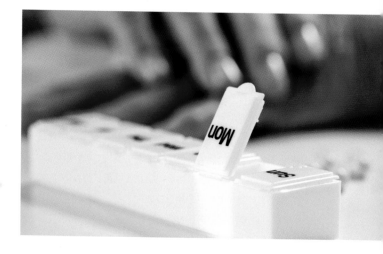

4 **GLP-1's given by injection.** These drugs work like your body's natural incretin hormones. They are much more potent than DPP-4 pills and, like DPP-4 pills, they rarely cause low blood sugar episodes. The drug names end in "tide" such as liraglutide (Victoza), exanatide (Bydureon), semaglutide (Ozempic) and dulaglutide (Trulicity). Victoza is a daily injection, whereas the other three are weekly. Recently, a version of semaglutide (Rybelsus) has been developed in pill form. If you have kidney disease or a high risk of heart disease or stroke, your doctor may prescribe one of these drugs.

A1C BENEFIT: Very Good to Excellent. **HYPOGLYCEMIA:** Rare. **WEIGHT:** Weight loss. ❤ Proven to reduce the risk of heart, blood vessel and kidney disease.

5 **SGLT2 Inhibitors.** These drugs take excess sugar from your blood and transport it to your urine. When there is extra sugar in the urine, a yeast or urinary tract infection is more common. These drug names end in "flozin" such as canagliflozin (Invokana), dapagliflozin (Farxiga), ertugliflozin (Steglatro) and empagliflozin (Jardiance). If you have heart disease, heart failure, or mild to moderate kidney disease, one of these drugs might be your doctor's choice for you. These drugs are one pill a day.

A1C BENEFIT: Very Good to Excellent. **HYPOGLYCEMIA:** Rare. **WEIGHT:** More weight loss. ❤ Proven to reduce the risk of heart, blood vessel and kidney disease.

SGLT2 Inhibitors transport extra sugar to your urine.

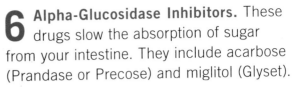

6 **Alpha-Glucosidase Inhibitors.** These drugs slow the absorption of sugar from your intestine. They include acarbose (Prandase or Precose) and miglitol (Glyset).

A1C BENEFIT: Fair. **HYPOGLYCEMIA:** Rare. **WEIGHT:** No weight change.

7 **TZD's.** These drugs help your insulin work better (they reduce insulin resistance). These drug names end in "zone" such as pioglitazone (Actos).

A1C BENEFIT: Very Good. **HYPOGLYCEMIA:** Rare. **WEIGHT:** More weight gain (mostly fluid).

8 **Weight Loss Agent (orlistat/Xenical).** With this drug you absorb less of the fat that you eat. This helps you lose some weight, which brings down blood sugar. It can give you stomach pain, diarrhea and urgency.

A1C BENEFIT: Good. **HYPOGLYCEMIA:** None. **WEIGHT:** More weight loss.

9 **Often, several diabetes medications work well together.** Different pills target different symptoms and protect different parts of your body. Ask about new pills that combine two different types of drugs into one pill. After being on one type of diabetes medication for years, it may lose its effect. Your doctor will try a new drug for three months, then check your A1C to see how well it works for you.

10 **Check the side effects listed for your medication.** Tell your doctor if you are having any side effects and ask about alternative medications.

Insulin

1 **Insulin is the most potent treatment for high blood sugar.** Drug companies produce various insulin products that mimic the human body's own insulin. Insulin is available in **1)** vials from which you inject it with a syringe, **2)** pen devices that connect to tiny pen needles, and **3)** a powder that you inhale.

2 **Basal insulin.** This type of insulin gives a fairly even effect for about 24 hours. It helps to manage sugar released at night from your liver. It is usually taken once a day, but may be taken twice a day. Basal insulin is often prescribed in combination with other diabetes medications.

3 **Mealtime insulin.** This type of insulin acts quickly to bring down the blood sugar rise after a meal. It lasts about two to four hours. Mealtime insulin is usually combined with basal insulin, since they work differently. The basal insulin reduces the amount of sugar the liver makes at night, while the mealtime insulin prevents the blood sugar from going up too high after eating.

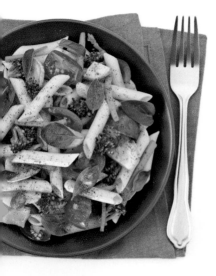

4 **The right dose for you.** When starting basal insulin, health care providers often prescribe a low dose. Over several weeks, the dose will be gradually increased based on your fasting blood sugar readings. This slow increase will reduce low blood sugar episodes and weight gain. Mealtime insulin can be dosed in different ways, but the dose usually depends on how many carbohydrates are in your meal and your blood sugar rise after eating. Many people are given a flexible dosing plan so that they may adjust the dose of mealtime insulin on their own with guidance from the health care team.

5 **The right time to take your insulin.** Most people take basal insulin in the morning or at bedtime, based on their own preferences and schedules. Being consistent with the time and not missing doses is very important. Mealtime insulin is usually taken just before eating. Depending on the insulin, it could be 15 minutes before the meal, just before eating, or even after finishing the last bite of food.

6 **Prepare for a low blood sugar episode.** Injected insulin can build up in your blood and cause a low blood sugar. When you feel the symptoms of a low blood sugar, your meter will read less than 70 mg/dL USA (4 mmol/L CAN). Immediately take 15 grams of glucose tablets or a tablespoon of sugar. See page 28 for a more complete list.

7 **Eat the right amount of food to match the insulin you are taking.** If you are only taking basal insulin, be consistent; eat similar-sized meals and snacks close to the same time every day. Using mealtime insulin gives you options to eat different-sized meals at different times and adjust the amount of insulin.

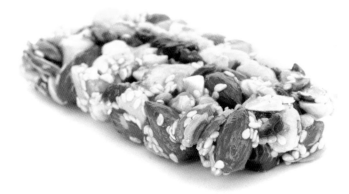

8 **Learn proper technique.** Talk to your nurse or pharmacist about how to properly inject and store your insulin. You can use an insulin pen, or use a needle with a syringe. Many people find the insulin pen easier to use. Inhaled insulin and insulin pumps are other ways you can take insulin that are becoming more popular.

With insulin pens, you no longer need to pinch the skin up like you would with a traditional insulin syringe needle.

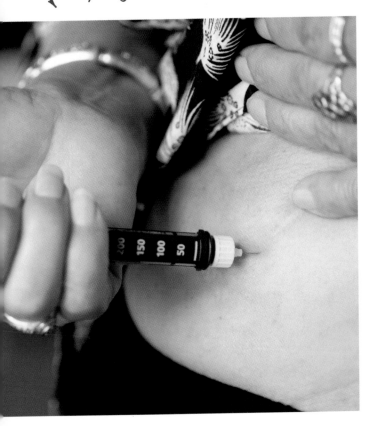

9 **Walk to help insulin work better.** If you take insulin every day, then it's best to walk every day too. Once you start walking more, the good news is that your insulin dose may be cut back. This will help prevent low blood sugar episodes. Carry glucose tablets when walking.

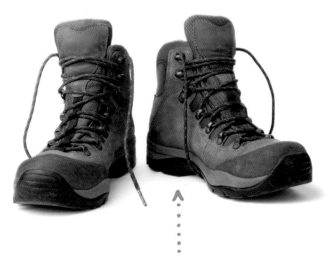

As you get fitter, you may want to go on a one- or two-hour walk or hike. Carry a water bottle, snacks, glucose tablets, cellphone and meter.

10 **What if insulin doesn't improve my blood sugar?** There are different types of insulin to try. Perhaps you need a combination of insulins or some other diabetes medication. Other ways to help improve your blood sugar include eating more fiber, sleeping better every night, and drinking water instead of juice or soft drinks.

Checking Your Sugar Level at Home

1 **Do I need to check?** Monitoring your blood sugar using a home device can help you and your health care team understand how well your medications, food choices and exercise are working. If you are on insulin or a diabetes medication that can cause low blood sugar episodes, checking is even more important. Some people may not need to check at all, or not more than a few times a month; others may need to check several times each day. Talk with your doctor or nurse to see how often you should check.

2 **Which meter to use?** Your pharmacist or diabetes educator can help you decide which meter is the easiest and the best buy for you. They will also show you how to use it. Most meters require you to prick your finger and put a drop of blood on a strip that is inserted into the meter. The newest kind of meter is called a continuous glucose monitor, or CGM. It is a patch with a computerized sensor placed on your arm. The sensor has a tiny filament that goes under your skin. The meter scans the patch to read your blood sugar.

3 **How much does a meter cost?** Ask your health insurer if they cover the costs of meters, strips and sensors. Some pharmacies have free meters, but costs for the strips or sensors can add up quickly.

4 **When should I check?** The best time to check your blood sugar is in the morning (fasting) and two hours after a meal. You may be advised to check at other times, especially if your insulin or medication needs to be adjusted. Always check when you feel you are having a low blood sugar episode. Checking before and after a meal or exercise can help you understand their effect on your blood sugar.

5 **What numbers should I be getting?** If you are newly diagnosed, it is best if your blood sugar level comes down gradually over several weeks.

Blood Sugar Targets Before and After Meals

FASTING OR BEFORE EATING:
Under 130 mg/dL USA (7 mmol/L CAN)

TWO HOURS AFTER EATING:
Under 180 mg/dL USA (10 mmol/L CAN)

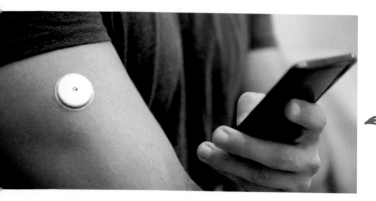

CGM is a good option if you need to know what your blood sugar is many times throughout the day and night.

6 What numbers should I be getting if I am elderly, or live alone, or have a heart condition, or have been having a lot of low blood sugars? Your doctor will want to keep your numbers higher than those noted in point 5. This reduces the risk of you having a low blood sugar episode, which can be an emergency situation.

7 What do I do with my numbers? At the time you check your blood sugar, write down what you ate, whether you exercised and any changes to your medication. Also, note your mood because emotions can affect your blood sugar levels. Now you can look for trends. Focus on the good numbers — what did you do to get these numbers? Many good phone apps can help you track your sugar readings and other data.

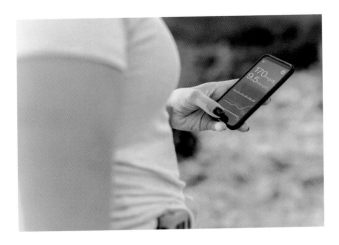

8 What are trends in my blood sugar level? A trend is a similar pattern over several days or a week. For example, you may notice that your sugar is low in the afternoon after a walk, or high in the evening after watching the news. A trend can help your doctor make the adjustments to your insulin or your medication to improve your blood sugar levels during the day and the night.

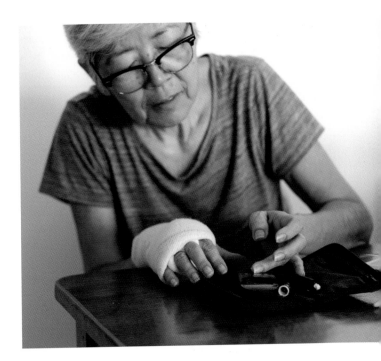

9 What does it mean when the meter reads HI (high)? Your blood sugar is about 540 mg/dL USA (30 mmol/L CAN) or more. **This means your sugar is so high that your meter can no longer read the level.** Right away recheck to make sure it was not an error. If the reading is still HI, call your doctor or seek help. Ask yourself what you did differently on this day or over the last few days. Do you have a cold or infection, or have you been in pain? Did you forget to take your insulin or diabetes pills? Have you been eating poorly and not walking?

10 What does it mean when the meter reads LO (low)? Your blood sugar is about 18 mg/dL USA (1 mmol/L CAN) or less. **This means your sugar is so low that your meter cannot detect any sugar.** There is no time to waste. Immediately eat 20 grams of glucose tablets or 4 teaspoons of sugar. Recheck right away to make sure it was not an error. Recheck in 15 minutes. If still low, treat with another 15 grams of glucose tablets. See pages 28–29 for more information.

Low Blood Sugar Episodes

1 **What does a low blood sugar feel like?** You may feel dizzy and weak, your hands can tremble, and you may start sweating especially on the back of your neck. People may notice you look pale. As your sugar drops lower you may get a headache or heart palpitations, and become confused and irritable. Your speech will slur and you will be unsteady when you walk or try to stand.

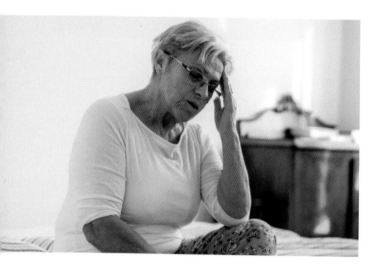

2 **What is the number for a low blood sugar?** 70 mg/dL USA (4 mmol/L CAN) or less on your blood glucose meter. A severe low is about 55 mg/dL (3 mmol/L) or less.

3 **What is the number for a low blood sugar if I am elderly or have a heart condition?** Your doctor may want you to keep your blood sugar at all times above 105 mg/dL USA (6 mmol/L CAN). Everyone needs an individualized goal from their doctor. If you are elderly, a low can happen more often, last longer and you may not have obvious symptoms.

4 **How to treat a low blood sugar?** Candy bars or food do not work fast enough. Take one of the following, which equal 15 grams of fast acting sugar. You will soon feel better. After 15 minutes if your meter still reads low, treat again.

- Fastest choice: 15 grams in total of glucose tablets (depending on the brand, this will be 3 to 5 tablets)

ALTERNATIVE CHOICES:
- 1 tablespoon sugar or honey
- 6 lifesavers
- ½ to ⅔ cup (125 to 150 mL) of juice or regular soft drink (diet soft drinks do not work!)

5 **What causes low blood sugar?** Either too much insulin or not enough carbohydrates.

6 **Why do you get a low blood sugar?** Here are examples of causes:
- your dose of insulin or diabetes medication is too strong
- by mistake, you took an extra dose of insulin or diabetes pills
- you missed a meal or snack
- you exercised or walked longer than usual
- you are sick, with diarrhea or vomiting
- you drank alcohol on an empty stomach

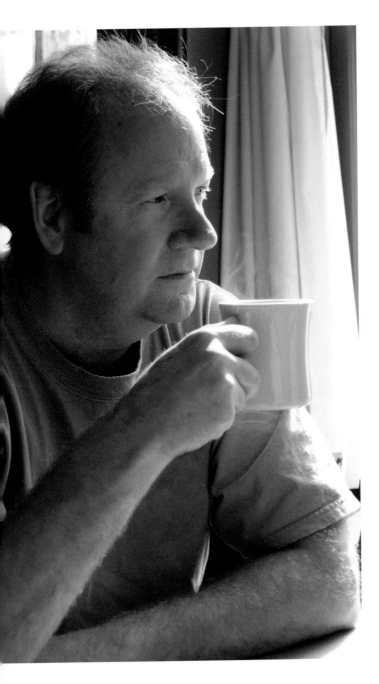

8 Prevent low blood sugar at night. A common cause of this is that your injected evening insulin is peaking in the night and moving sugar out of your blood. Recommendations might include:

- reduce the amount of insulin you take for up to five days, then reassess
- change to a longer acting basal insulin
- change the time you take your insulin
- have a small snack before bedtime
- use a continuous glucose monitor that has an alarm

9 What if I feel low but my meter tells me I am normal or high? Two things can cause this:

1. A fast drop in your blood sugar can make you feel low. For example, if you just went for a vigorous walk it could drop from 250 to 150 mg/dL USA (14 to 8 mmol/L CAN).
2. A gradual drop in your blood sugar to a more normal level, one that your body is not used to.

Either way, you are not experiencing a real blood sugar low, just a shift in blood sugar level. If you feel really unwell, have a couple of Tic Tacs, which equals only 1 gram of carbohydrate. The best advice is to rest and drink water.

7 Prevent low blood sugar. If you see a trend where your readings are low every day, you must talk with your doctor or diabetes educator about your diet and exercise. Here are changes they might suggest:

- reduce your insulin or diabetes pills
- change the time that you take them
- change the combination of your medications

10 Safety first. Do not drive or operate machinery when your blood sugar is low. This can be just as risky as if you were impaired. If you have any doubts, check your blood sugar before you get behind the wheel. Always have glucose tablets handy.

Reduce a High Morning Blood Sugar

1 Hormones affect morning (fasting) blood sugar. Your blood sugar naturally drops through the night when you are not eating. Once it gets so low, around dawn, hormones such as cortisol and glucagon activate the liver to release stored sugar into your bloodstream. This helps wake you up. Insulin is then released to bring the blood sugar down. If you have diabetes these hormones are often not working properly and the blood sugar remains high in the morning.

2 Take metformin. A diabetes pill called metformin (Glucophage or Glumetza) helps stop the liver from releasing sugar into the blood in the early dawn hours. Your dose may need to be increased to the maximum to work for you. It can take a week or two to see a difference.

3 Add other medications. In addition to metformin, your doctor may add other medications to reduce the hormone glucagon so the liver will release less sugar. The types of medications known as GLP-1's and TZD's help in this manner. SGLT2 inhibitors also reduce high fasting sugar by transporting the extra sugar from the blood into the urine. Please see the Diabetes Medications page.

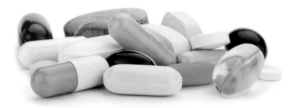

4 Change in basal insulin. Basal insulin acts evenly throughout the night to help you wake up with a good blood sugar level. It is the most potent treatment for high morning sugar. If you are taking a basal insulin and the morning sugar is still high, talk to your health care team. Your dose may have to be adjusted.

5 Get a good night's sleep. If you do not sleep soundly, stress hormones will raise your blood sugar overnight and into the morning. Darken your room for a sound sleep. Turn off all electronics half an hour before bed. If you have pain that is keeping you awake, talk to your doctor about taking a longer-acting pain medication before bed. Ask your doctor if you need to be tested for a condition called obstructive sleep apnea, which affects many people with diabetes.

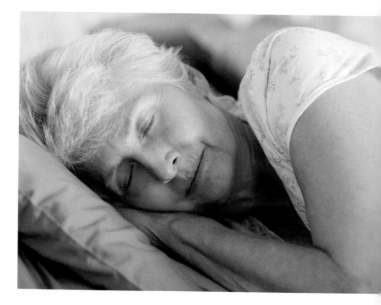

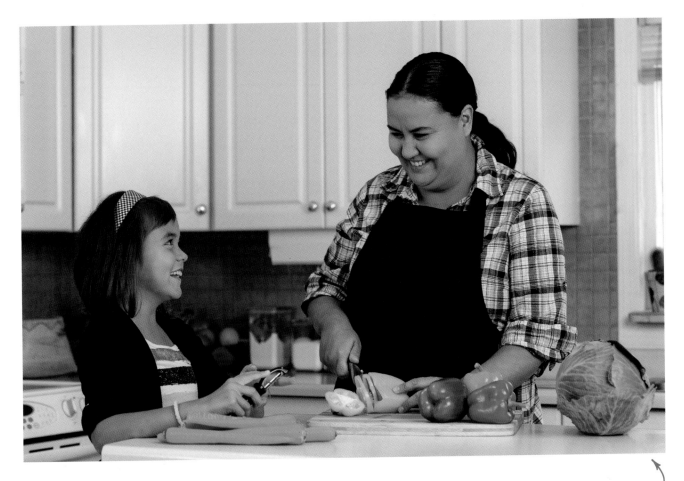

6 **Eat a small breakfast.** This encourages the insulin to start working, which brings down your blood sugar. Choose foods that are high in fiber. Include some protein or a small amount of fat.

7 **Walk during the day or after dinner.** Exercise helps your insulin work better and brings down blood sugar. This benefit can last 12 to 18 hours, right through to the next morning.

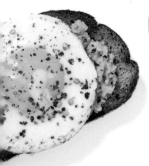

Recommended walking shoes for those with diabetes have a deep toe box.

8 **Eat a small dinner meal.** When you eat a large dinner meal that is high in carbohydrates, your blood sugar rises to a high level and can still be high the next morning.

9 **Be careful with evening snacks.** With the right dose of insulin, most people do not need an evening snack to prevent low blood sugar at night. If you are hungry, try snacks that are high in fiber and protein, but not too high in carbohydrates.

10 **Lose five to ten pounds.** Weight loss soon after diagnosis can help your hormones return to a more stable level. Plus, this weight loss when kept off can reduce the development of complications later.

Sick Day Advice

1 **Make a sick day plan before you get sick.** Your doctor or health care provider can help you with your plan. Write this information down and put it into this section of the book — and let your family know where it is.

2 **Continue to take your insulin and diabetes medication when sick.** This is because the stress of being ill usually makes blood sugar rise. Your doctor will tell you if you need to stop any meds. Ask what cold, flu or pain medications are safe for you, including cough drops and cough syrups.

3 **If you live alone, let a family member or friend know you are sick.** They can call you and visit you until you feel better.

4 **If you have a meter, check your blood sugar at least every four hours.** This will help you see any changes. If you have a low blood sugar episode, treat it and keep checking. To reduce lows or highs, your doctor may adjust your insulin or medications.

5 **Drink sugar-free fluids every hour that you are awake.** Warm water or broth soothes a sore throat, while cold water helps cool a fever. Gatorade Zero and Powerade Zero help replace lost nutrients due to diarrhea or vomiting. Try a cup of ginger tea to reduce feelings of nausea.

6 **Eat a little to keep up your energy.** Have a small glass of juice; a meal replacement drink like Boost; a scoop of ice cream or a small yogurt; rice pudding; a small banana; a piece of toast; a few crackers with cheese; or a bowl of chicken noodle soup.

7 **If you cannot keep food down.** If you have diarrhea or are vomiting, your blood sugar could quickly drop too low. Keep drinking fluids and check your blood sugar more often. Your doctor may suggest you temporarily cut back your mealtime insulin or other diabetes medications.

8 **Call your doctor or a medical help line or go to a clinic or emergency room if:**
- your blood sugar stays at 300 mg/dL USA (15 mmol/L CAN) or higher for two or more readings
- you have one low blood sugar after another even though you are treating them
- you have severe vomiting, diarrhea or fever
- you are very thirsty, have muscle cramps, confusion and dark pee (these symptoms, together, may indicate dehydration)
- there is blood in your urine
- you feel numb or stiff in any part of your body
- your symptoms get worse
- you have unusual symptoms or you are unsure and need further advice

9 **Call 911.** For anything more severe, including trouble breathing and shortness of breath, chest pain, seizure or fainting.

10 **Keep warm and rest.** Wrap yourself in a favorite blanket and go to bed.

Lose Five Pounds and Keep It Off

1 **Know what you eat.** For a couple of days, write down what you eat, how much you eat and when you eat. Get to know you and the reasons you eat.

2 **To get started, set small realistic goals and you will feel good about yourself.** Here are a few examples:
- I will walk 15 minutes three days a week
- I will eat two vegetables every day
- I will not eat potato chips on the weekend

3 **Drink water.** Drink fewer sugary drinks and drink less alcohol.

4 **Clean out your kitchen cupboards, fridge and freezer.** The more junk food, sugary drinks and alcohol you have at home, the more of them you will eat and drink.

5 **Open the front door, not the fridge door.** Walking and other exercise uses calories you have already eaten.

6 **Don't eat after 9:00 pm.** After your last evening snack — and keep it small — brush your teeth and have a drink of water.

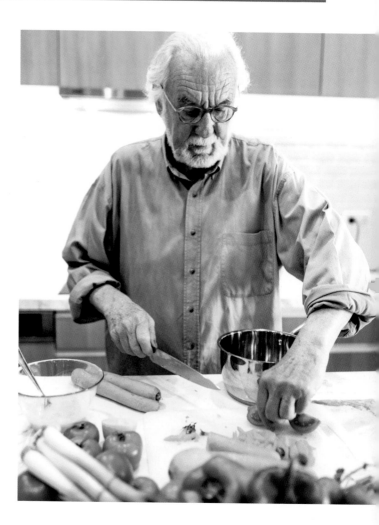

7 **Eat home-cooked meals.** You will most likely be a healthier weight. This is true whether you live alone or with your family.

8 **Enjoy treats once in a while.** Have a favorite food or dessert now and again. What's most important is your long-term goal to be healthy.

9 **Connect with others.** Finding new friends with healthy habits can be an exciting change.

Try a fun class like Zumba. You can help each other stay on track and keep up your new healthy habits together!

10 **Rapid weight gain is a medical emergency.** Doctors say that if you quickly gain five or more pounds due to short-term overeating, treat this as a medical emergency that needs to be dealt with right away. It is easiest to lose extra weight in the first few weeks after you have gained it. Don't delay.

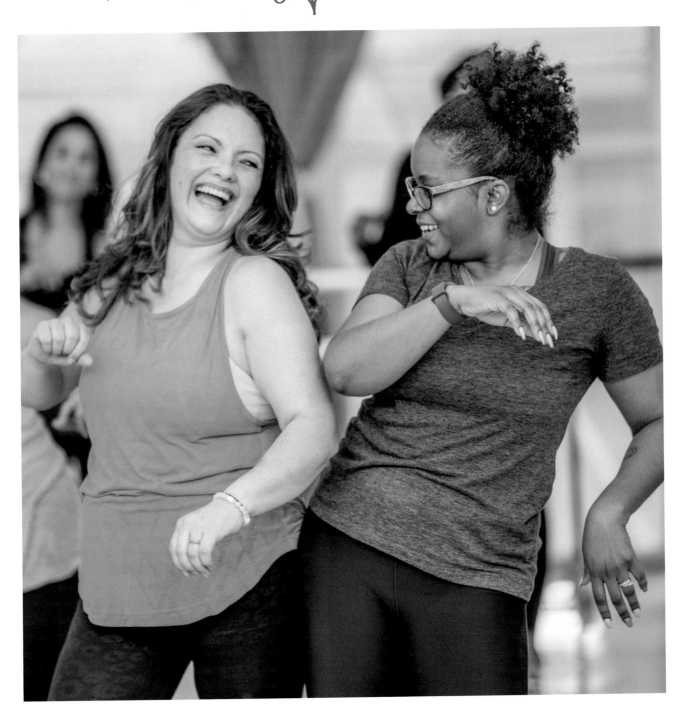

How to Gain Weight if You Are Underweight

1 I am thin, why did I get diabetes?
If you are 70 years or older, your pancreas may no longer make enough insulin. Or you may have a strong family history of diabetes, be a smoker, or have high blood pressure or high triglycerides.

2 I am thin, why do I keep losing weight?
High blood sugar and a lack of insulin can cause weight loss. The lack of insulin means the extra sugar builds up in your blood and eventually leaves the body through urine. This loss of sugar (calories) is one common reason for your weight loss.

3 You may need diabetes medication to help you gain weight. This is especially true if your blood sugar is consistently high. Medication or injected insulin will help your body absorb sugar and even other nutrients that help you gain muscle and weight.

4 Have three small meals each day, plus snacks. This spreads carbohydrates and calories out during the day, which makes it easier for your body to absorb the calories.

5 Eat more protein. Such as meat, chicken and fish; peanut butter and nuts and seeds; and beans and lentils.

6 Add more fat and oil. Extra margarine, butter, oils and even avocado can be added to salads, soups, mashed potatoes, rice, pasta and scrambled eggs.

7 Eat more dairy foods. These are good to keep your bones strong and give you protein. Drink regular or lactose-free milk, or unsweetened soy milk — choose whole or 2% milk. Cheese is nourishing, as are yogurts that are 2% to 7% fat. Please note that almond milk, cashew milk and rice milk are low in protein; they are not recommended for weight gain.

8 Double the protein in your milk. Add ¼ cup (60 mL) of skim milk powder or commercial protein supplement to a cup (250 mL) of milk in a container with a tight lid. Shake it well and let it sit overnight in the fridge to dissolve fully. You can drink this milk as it is or use it on breakfast cereals or to make pancakes or puddings.

9 Diabetes meal replacement drinks. If your appetite is low these are easy to drink. Start with one a day or split one into two snacks in a day. Examples are Glucerna, Boost Diabetic and Ensure Diabetes. They provide protein and slow-release carbohydrates to prevent peaks in blood sugar.

10 **Keep active.** A 15-minute walk will help improve your appetite. Walking strengthens your bones and helps you put weight on more evenly.

How People Improve Their Blood Sugar

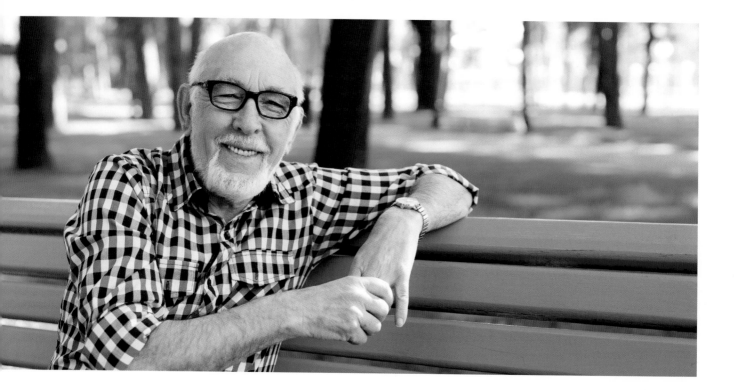

1 **Be kind to yourself.** Think positive thoughts about yourself, learn ways to relax and sleep well. Positive hormones are known to improve blood sugar levels.

2 **Start your diabetes medication.** Your doctor will likely start you on metformin. You will feel positive when you see your blood sugar numbers come down.

3 **Treat infections.** An infection causes your blood sugar level to rise. After the infection clears, blood sugar will improve.

4 **Manage pain caused by diabetes.** Use cushioned shoes, medicated creams and doctor-recommended pain pills. Try deep breathing exercises and gentle massage to relax.

5 **Check your blood sugar.** If you see a high blood sugar count, you may be motivated to eat less at your next meal and go for a short walk.

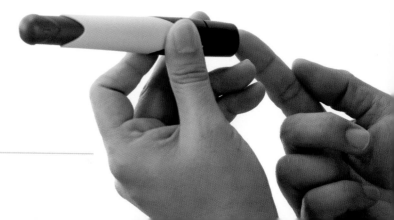

6 **Change any medication that makes you hungry.** Ask your pharmacist about this side effect. Certain drugs, such as some antidepressants, diabetes pills and insulin can make you feel hungry.

7 **Make regular appointments.** Phone or visit a nurse, dietitian or diabetes educator at a diabetes center. They can answer your questions and explain your lab results. However, the best benefit is their personal support for you. They know how much work it takes to make changes.

8 **No fad diets.** You can quickly lose weight on a fad diet, but most people gain the weight back. You want slow, long-term changes and improvements in your weight and blood sugar.

9 **No more soft drinks.** This can make a huge difference in the amount of daily sugar you consume. Let your friends know your progress, "One week and no Coke!"

10 **Walk every day.** Exercise helps insulin work well to remove extra sugar from your blood. Start with a 15-minute walk. You will begin to feel so much better.

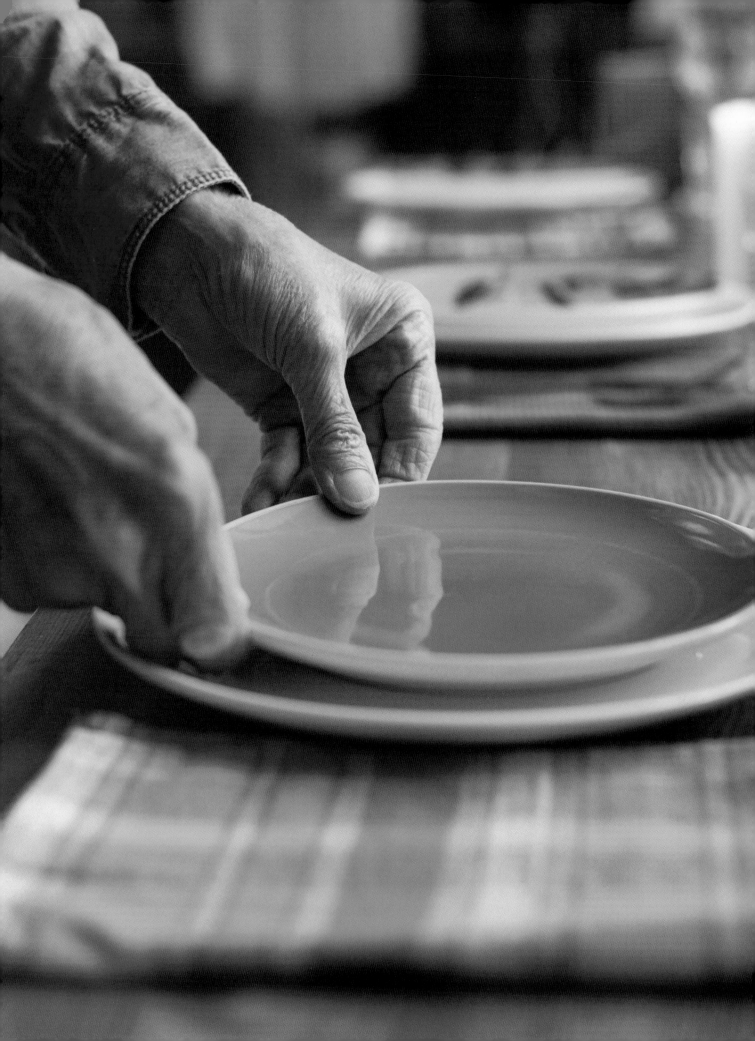

Set the Table

Mindful Eating

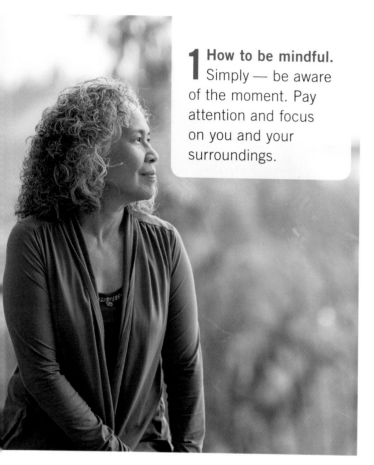

1 How to be mindful. Simply — be aware of the moment. Pay attention and focus on you and your surroundings.

2 Mindful eating. Take time to look at your food. Taste each mouthful. Respect the healthy nutrition in the food. Enjoy the feeling of eating.

3 Balance your cravings. Cravings can lead to unhealthy eating habits. Try these mindful eating ways: **D**elay, Breathe **D**eeply, **D**rink Water and **D**istract Yourself.

4 Delay. Give yourself time to think. Ask yourself are you really hungry? When did you last eat? How much did you eat? Think about what you are craving and the reasons.

5 Breathe Deeply. Sit down and close your eyes. Breathe slowly in and out. Feel calm and pay attention to your body's needs.

6 Drink Water. You may just be thirsty. Water is essential for every function in your body. We often need water more than we need food.

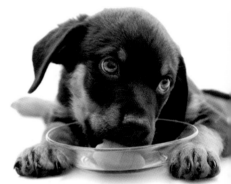

7 Distract Yourself. Leave the kitchen. There is always a household chore or something else to do.

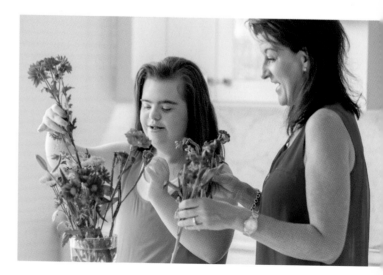

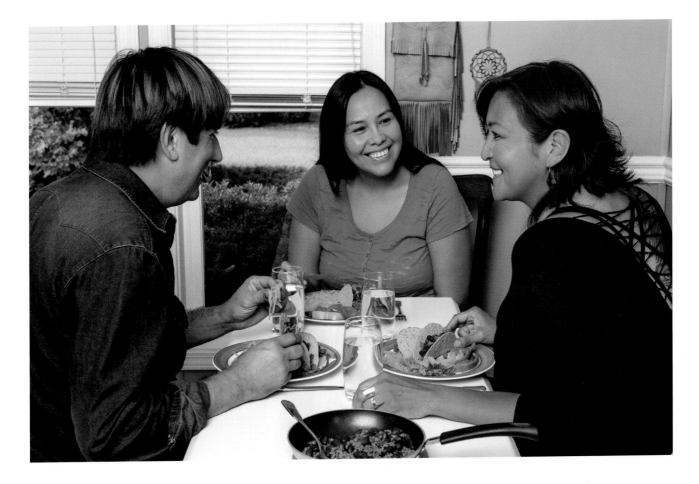

8 **Eat at a table.** This is where family gathers. Give thanks and share stories. Even if you eat alone, set a nice table and treat each meal as a ceremony.

9 **It takes practice.** Mindful eating is positive thinking and action. Think about the food before you eat, not after you eat, because then it's too late. Then you may have negative thoughts about your weight.

10 **A mindfulness exercise.** Focus for one minute while you are sitting or standing still in your house or outside. Count how many different sounds you hear in that minute.

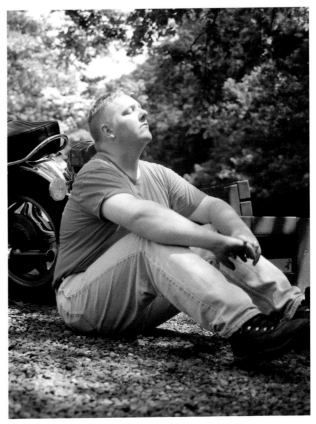

Portion Control Secrets

1 Use your own hand to measure portions. The hand guide below works for your own body size. Use hand portions and you will eat less food.

2 Serve food in the kitchen. Large plates of food on the table can tempt you to eat second or third helpings.

3 Use smaller bowls and plates. You will serve smaller portions of food. Usually it's just the right amount. We have become used to an overabundance of food served to us at restaurants.

4 Fill up half your plate with vegetables. More vegetables means less room for meat and potatoes.

5 Set your table with water glasses for every meal. Even for breakfast. We lose water during sleep just from breathing. Replenish with water; it is better than juice.

6 Have a small mid-afternoon snack. This way you won't be so hungry at dinnertime. Try a piece of cheese, 10 pecan or walnut halves, a cup of chai tea or a "lite" brand of cocoa made with milk.

DINNER MEAL PORTIONS

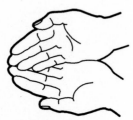

Fill your hands with vegetables and fruits

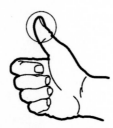

An end-of-thumb portion of oil, fat, butter or margarine; an end-of-thumb portion of sugar

1 to 2 fist-size portions of starch (rice, bread, grains, potatoes)

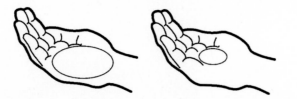

Protein: A palm-size portion of chicken, meat, fish, eggs, beans or lentils OR half a palm-size portion of nuts, seeds or cheese

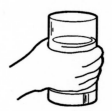

Drink water with every meal

7 Don't eat directly from the original food package. Instead, portion only smaller amounts of foods such as chips, cookies, ice cream and candy into small bowls. Put the rest away in the cupboard.

8 Out of sight — out of mind. Put away foods that tempt you — or better yet, don't buy them.

9 Eat fewer salty, sugary and fried foods. These foods create cravings you want to avoid. We tend to eat larger portions of the foods we crave.

10 See life-size photos of meals and snacks showing the correct portions. These are found in the second and third book in this series (see page 192).

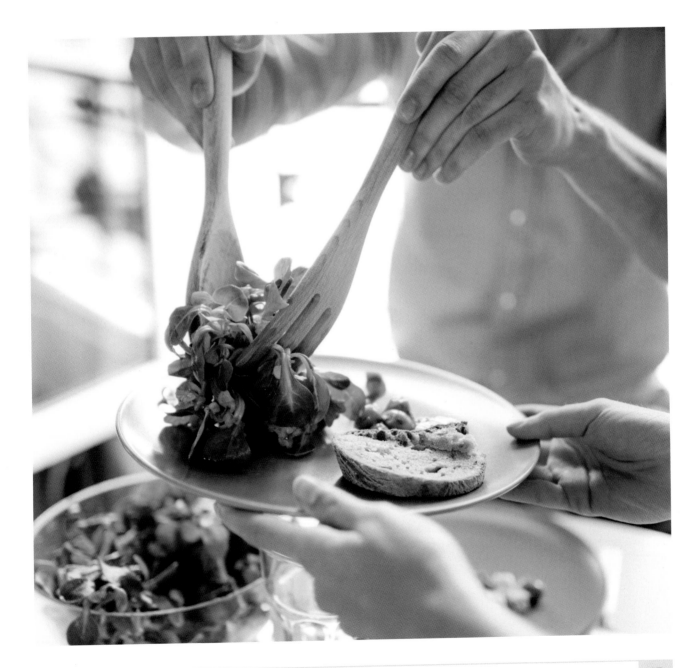

More Vegetables on the Table

1 Double-up veggies. Make a new rule — two or more vegetables at your main meal. Serve them on the side, or add extra fresh, frozen or canned vegetables into recipes.

2 Vegetables have healing power. Eat vegetables of various colors to help manage diabetes and its complications. Each vegetable has its own blend of vitamins, minerals and phytochemicals.

3 Make vegetable stock. Use extra vegetables from the garden and vegetables from your fridge before they go bad. Boil until mushy, then discard the vegetables. Cool the stock and freeze in containers to use later in soups, gravies and sauces.

4 Make the vegetable the star of the meal. Cut a bell pepper or squash in half and remove the seeds. Stuff it with a vegetarian or meat sauce, or beans and rice, and bake it in the oven. Instead of a taco or tortilla shell, use a large piece of iceberg or romaine lettuce and make a lettuce wrap.

5 Include a vegetable at breakfast! Before cooking, grate raw carrots into oatmeal. Have sliced cucumbers or tomatoes on the side with your egg. Make a vegetable omelet.

Next week, try one new vegetable! ---→

6 **Vegetable-based smoothies, occasionally.** Blended vegetables lose much of their healthful whole fiber, but they keep all their vitamins and minerals. An easy recipe is $\frac{1}{2}$ to 1 cup of raw spinach, $\frac{1}{4}$ small avocado, $\frac{1}{3}$ cup milk, $\frac{1}{3}$ cup plain yogurt, and 1 tsp lemon juice. Blend till smooth.

7 **Salads with or without lettuce.** Salads can be made with salad greens or try raw vegetables. Chop green, yellow and red peppers with a sprinkle of feta cheese. Chop broccoli, cauliflower and apple. Add your favorite salad dressing.

Enjoy coleslaw!

8 **Snacks on the go.** Eat mini carrots and mini cucumbers. An old favorite is still great, celery with Cheez Whiz or peanut butter. Veggies with dip are always popular.

9 **Buy local farm produce.** Grocery stores provide us with fresh vegetables all year round. In most communities you can buy local produce in the summer through fall, for the freshest flavor at a good price.

10 **Grow your own veggies.** If you do not consider yourself a gardener, plant a couple of zucchini or cucumber seeds in a warm sunny spot. Buy a cherry tomato plant for your garden or in a pot. Visit garden centers and ask which vegetables grow best in your climate. If you do not have the space for a garden, ask about community gardens in your area.

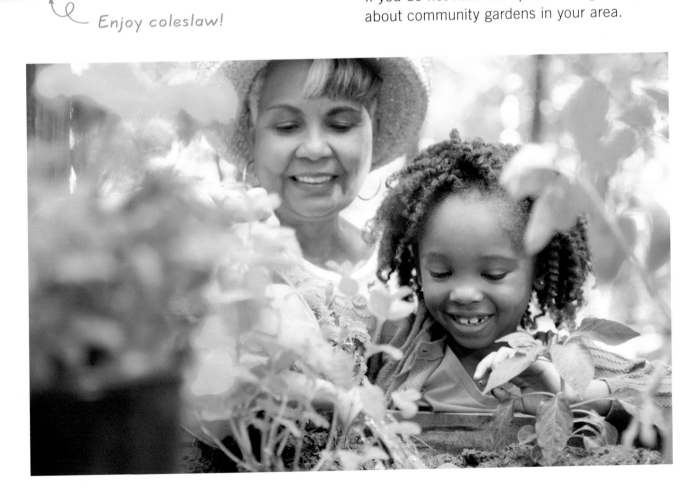

Diabetes Super Foods

Breakfast Foods

1 **Oats and Oatmeal.*** High in soluble fiber and a great way to start your day.

SUPER NUTRIENT **Avenanthramide:** This antioxidant is only found in oats. It increases blood flow to help lower blood pressure.

2 **Oranges, Apples and Bananas.*** All fruits are healthy. These three are affordable and, as an environmental bonus, are not plastic wrapped.

SUPER NUTRIENTS **Vitamin C, Fiber and Potassium:** Oranges are rich in vitamin C that can help wounds heal. Apples are an excellent source of fiber. Bananas have potassium to help lower blood pressure.

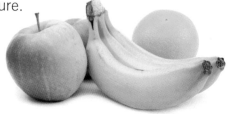

3 **Almonds and Peanuts.*** Slice and chop them; sprinkle them on your breakfast cereal. Peanut butter is classic spread on toast.

SUPER NUTRIENT **Magnesium:** It may help improve fasting blood sugar because it increases insulin sensitivity (helps insulin work better).

4 **Yogurt and Milk.*** Plain yogurt and low-fat milk are nutrient boosters at any meal.

SUPER NUTRIENTS **Calcium and added Vitamin D:** They are good for our teeth and bones. Research also shows calcium has a role in healthy weight and healthy blood pressure. Vitamin D has been shown to decrease insulin resistance.

Lunch Foods

5 **Dark Greens.** Spinach, romaine lettuce, asparagus and green peas. Add cooked asparagus to a wrap or add a handful of frozen green peas to a soup.

SUPER NUTRIENT **Folic Acid:** By helping to reduce a chemical called homocysteine, it may reduce your risk for heart attack and stroke.

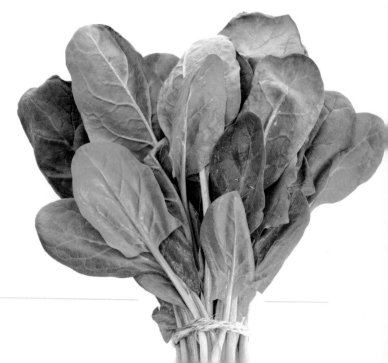

6 Avocados. Enjoy in salads and in sandwiches and wraps.

SUPER NUTRIENT Monounsaturated Fat: This fat may lower your "bad" cholesterol level and raise your "good" cholesterol. This may reduce your risk for a heart attack or stroke.

7 Legumes.* Such as lentils, kidney beans and chickpeas. Canned legumes and beans are ready-to-eat; dried ones take longer but are very affordable.

SUPER NUTRIENT Plant Protein: When plant protein replaces meat protein there is less stress on your kidneys. This is especially important if you have reduced kidney function.

Dinner Foods

8 Fish. From a can, or cooked from fresh or frozen, fish can be added to a wrap or sandwich, or served for a main meal, or raw in sushi.

SUPER NUTRIENT Omega-3 Fat: Found especially in cold water fish like salmon, trout and sardines. This fat is healthy for your brain and eyes. Research shows it may lower your risk for heart attacks and stroke as it lowers triglycerides (blood fat) and it reduces blood clots.

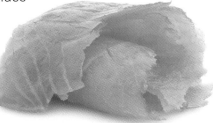

9 Converted and Long Grain Rice.* This includes converted rice (also called parboiled) such as Uncle Ben's Original Converted Rice, long grain rice (brown or white) and basmati rice.

SUPER NUTRIENT Amylose (a resistant starch): The rices named above have more amylose than other rice does. This gives them a lower glycemic index than other kinds of rice, meaning your blood sugar doesn't rise as quickly.

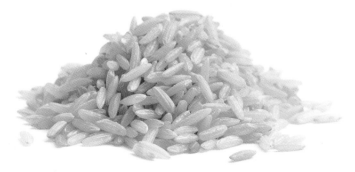

10 Cruciferous Vegetables. Such as broccoli, cauliflower, turnip, cabbage, bok choy, Brussels sprouts, kale and radishes. Grown and eaten worldwide, they are now staples in North American grocery stores.

SUPER NUTRIENT Sulforaphane: This antioxidant can reduce inflammation in blood vessels and helps protect against diabetes-related blood vessel damage.

Try the delicious Broccoli Cheese Soup on page 79.

*Contains carbohydrate — eat in moderation.

Low Glycemic Eating

1 **Glycemic index (GI) of carbohydrates.** Carbohydrates are all starches, sugars and fiber foods. The glycemic index is the time it takes after eating different carbohydrates to raise your blood sugar.

2 **Glycemic load of a meal.** This depends on both the GI of the food and the quantity you eat. It affects how quickly and how much your blood sugar rises after the meal.

3 **Low and high GI carbohydrates.** Low GI carbohydrates are slowly digested, so they raise your blood sugar slowly. High GI carbohydrates enter the bloodstream quickly and you can get a high spike in your blood sugar.

4 **What are low GI carbohydrates?** These foods, which have lots of fiber, include vegetables and most fruits; whole grain foods; beans, lentils and split peas; barley, bulgur, quinoa and buckwheat; oats, long grain rice and converted rice. These foods can take 30 minutes or more to raise your blood sugar.

5 **Raw plant foods are low GI.** They take longer to chew and digest, and have lots of fiber. At breakfast, spoon some raw oatmeal into your yogurt; include fresh fruit at lunch and raw vegetables at dinner.

6 **What are high GI carbohydrates?** White and brown sugar, honey and syrup, on their own or added to foods, and sodas and sweets are your biggest source. Fruit juice is a high GI food because the fiber has been removed or finely chopped. High GI also includes white foods like white bread, short grain white rice, instant noodles, plain soda crackers and white pasta. All these foods raise your blood sugar in five to 15 minutes.

7 **Tip to slow down high GI carbohydrates.** Eat them with a small amount of protein or fat. For instance, cheese or peanut butter are the proteins, and crackers or white bread are the carbohydrates.

8 **Lemon or vinegar can slow down carbs.** Add to any meal from salads to stews. Mix in just before eating to boost flavor.

9 **Tip to reduce glycemic load of a meal.** Since portion size is involved, make a goal to eat less. Until then, take a walk after large meals to reduce blood sugar.

10 **Eating too much protein and fat can raise blood sugar.** Digestion is complex. If you eat a large amount of meat or fat at a meal, especially at a low-carb meal, the body has a way to convert these foods into sugars and you may get a rise in your blood sugar.

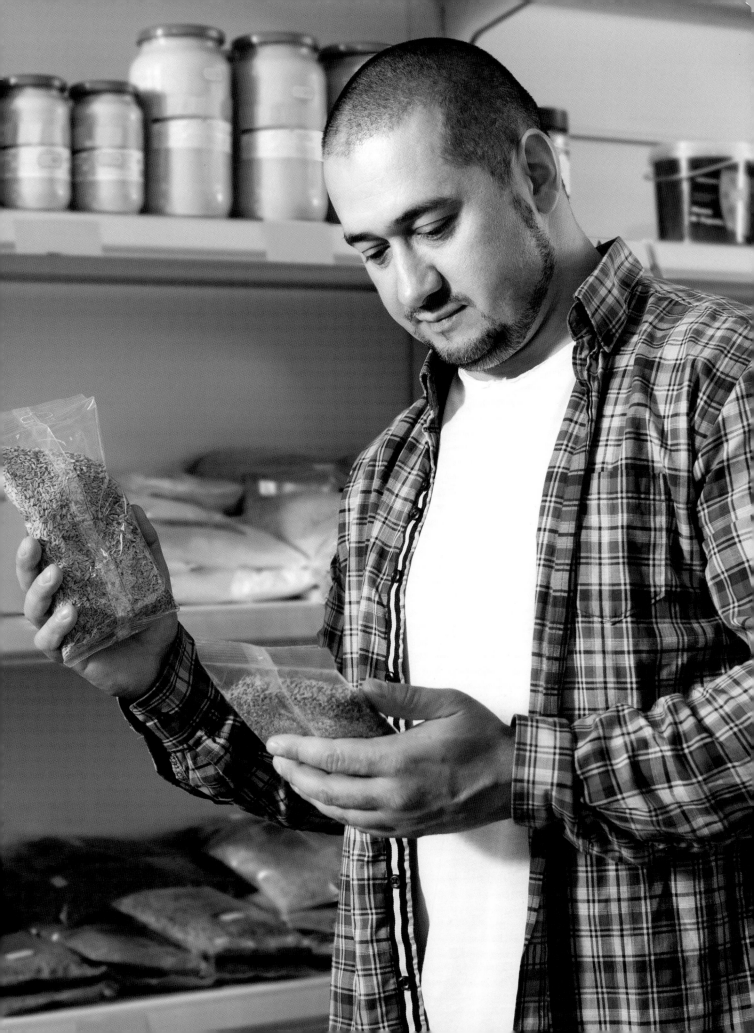

Eat Less Processed Food

1 **Set a goal.** Review the processed foods listed on these pages. Every month make it your goal to eat or drink less of a processed food or drink.

2 **Restaurant meals.** Pizzas, burgers, fried chicken, fries, cake and ice cream are all highly addictive processed foods.

3 **Soft drinks and sweet drinks.** Colas are linked to the rise in diabetes around the world. Sweet drinks include all juices, sports drinks, energy drinks and iced teas. Many cans and plastic bottles end up in the ocean and landfill as garbage.

4 **Super-sweetened hot and iced coffees and teas.** At the drive-through or standing in line, the flashing ads influence us to buy super-sweetened, and often super-sized, drinks and snacks. This is an opportunity to say "no."

This large drink can have up to 300 calories and 11 teaspoons (44 grams) of sugar!

5 **Potato chips, Cheezies, nacho chips.** Avoid the tempting chip aisle when grocery shopping.

TOO MUCH FAT!

TOO MUCH SUGAR!

PSST...
Check out
the recipe
on page 93
for a fried
chicken
alternative!

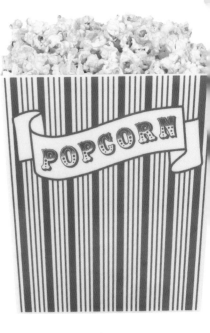

6 Movie popcorn. The large bag of buttered movie theatre popcorn has 1,400 calories and a teaspoon of salt!

When watching a movie at home enjoy a lighter popcorn option, see page 110.

see page 110

7 Store-bought cakes, cookies, muffins, pies, donuts and sweetened breakfast cereals. These processed foods are loaded with fat and sugar.

8 Luncheon meat, bacon, wieners and sausages. These processed foods are loaded with salt, fat and preservatives.

9 Canned foods, packaged soups and instant noodles. These processed foods have a large amount of salt added.

10 Big-size (300 gram) chocolate bars. Two generations ago, people were satisfied with an occasional chocolate bar that weighed about 50 grams.

Craving chocolate? Choose an occasional 50 g bar. Don't put this big one in your cart.

Read Food Labels

1 **Each food package has an Ingredients list and a Nutrition Facts table.** Comparing the labels of similar foods can help you make the healthiest choices.

2 **Ingredients are listed in order from the most to the least.** The list includes everything in the package: food items and also any preservatives, flavoring or added vitamins.

Sample Ingredients list and Nutrition Facts table for granola cereal:

Ingredients: Rolled oats, rolled whole wheat, brown sugar, modified milk ingredients, dried unsweetened coconut, coconut oil, corn syrup, almonds, honey, natural flavour.

Nutrition Facts
Per 2/3 Cup (45 g)

Amount Per Serving	% Daily Value
Calories 215	
Fat 8 g	6%
Saturated 6 g	28%
+ Trans 0 g	
Cholesterol 0 mg	0%
Sodium 35 mg	1%
Carbohydrate 32 g	10%
Fibre 4 g	15%
Sugars 10 g	
Protein 5 g	
Vitamin A	0%
Vitamin C	0%
Calcium	2%
Iron	8%

3 **The Nutrition Facts table lists the total nutrients from all the items in this food.** So when you eat the serving size of 2/3 cup of granola, you will get 6 grams of saturated fat, 35 mg of sodium, 4 grams of fiber, and so on. Your dietitian can look at the Nutrition Facts table and Ingredients list together and match things up for you. For example, the saturated fat comes from the dried coconut and the coconut oil.

4 **Serving size.** This is at the top of the Nutrition Facts table. For example, per 2/3 cup cereal or per 1 slice of bread. If the label lists per 1 cup, and you eat 2 cups, then you double the calories and other nutrients.

5 **Calories.** Often, when comparing products, your best choice is the one with the fewest calories per serving.

6 **Fat — Saturated.** This type of fat, which comes from animals and hydrogenated palm oils, should be limited.
5 GRAMS OF FAT = 1 TEASPOON

7 **Sodium.** The less sodium, the better.
30% SODIUM = ONE THIRD OF DAILY VALUE

8 **Carbohydrate — Fiber.** The more fiber, the better.

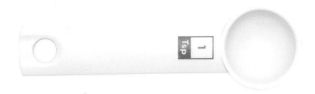

9 Carbohydrate — Sugars. The less sugar, the better.

4 GRAMS OF SUGAR = 1 TEASPOON

10 Food labels list a wide range of items, depending on the product. Look for vitamins, minerals and healthy fats such as monounsaturated fat and omega-3 fat. And remember, some of the best foods — fresh fruits and vegetables — have no labels at all!

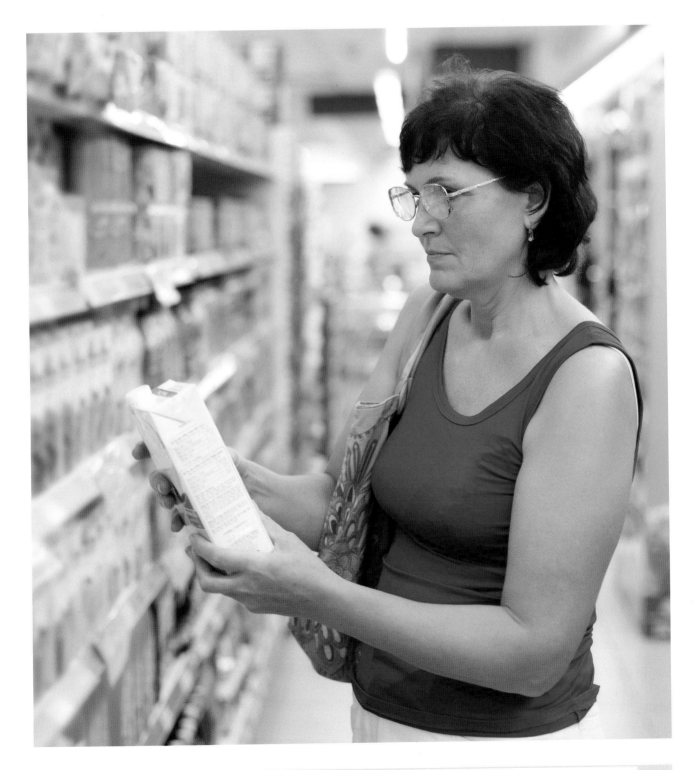

Everyday Cereals and Dessert Cereals

Say Yes to Everyday Cereals

1 Oatmeal. The soluble fiber in oatmeal and oat bran helps remove the bad cholesterol (LDL) from your blood. (See page 20.) Try overnight oatmeal: soak raw oatmeal overnight in an equal amount of milk plus some berries or sliced fruit and you can add a teaspoon of chia seeds or flax seeds.

2 Other cooked cereals. Cream of Wheat is an excellent source of iron. Choose the original variety rather than the instant. Fiber-rich cereals include grits (coarsely ground cornmeal) and flax-based cereals like Sunny Boy and Red River.

3 All-Bran, Bran Buds, Grape-Nuts and Fiber One. These cereals have some added sugar but are a great source of fiber, B vitamins and zinc. A great way to start your morning.

4 Dry cereals with a good amount of fiber and zero added sugar, fat or salt. Shredded wheat is a great choice.

5 Other healthy cold cereals. Check the label. Per cup (250 mL), there should be 3 g or more of fiber, 4 g or less of sugar, and 2 g or less of fat. Examples are Cheerios, Wheaties, All-Bran Flakes and no-sugar-added muesli.

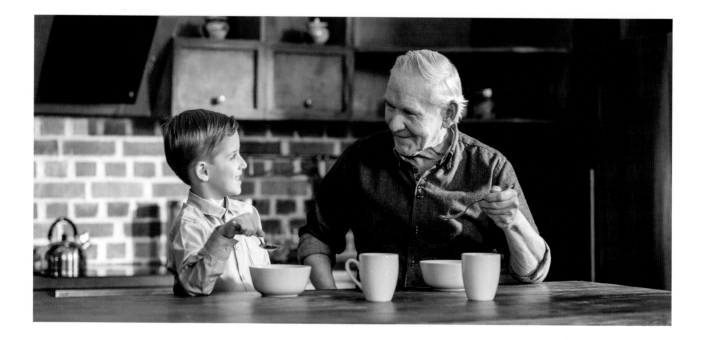

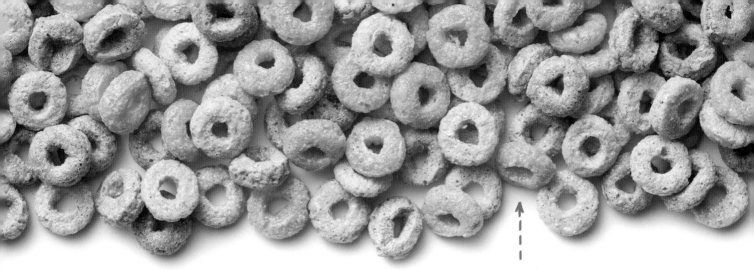

Too much sugar.

Say No to Dessert Cereals

6 **Sweetened breakfast cereals are really dessert.** Most brands have more sugar than grain.

7 **Honey and frosted cereals.** Per 1 cup, these typically have 3 teaspoons (12 g) of sugar or more.

8 **Granola.** Some brands of granola have three times as many calories and sugar as oatmeal and eight times as much fat.

Check the label. Look for granola brands with more oats and less sugar and fat.

9 **Deceptive ads on cereal boxes.** The "Multi Grain" version of Cheerios is advertised as high in grains and good for the heart. But per cup (250 mL), it has an additional teaspoon of sugar and similar fiber, compared to regular Cheerios.

10 **Still want sweetened cereal?** Make it your dessert and sprinkle sweetened cereal over plain yogurt. Or, sprinkle it over the healthy everyday cereal.

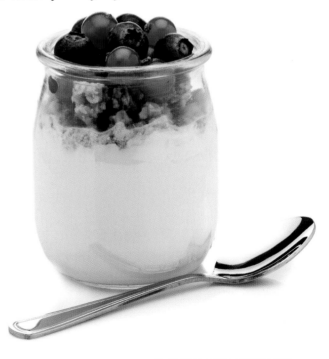

Worst Beverages for Diabetes

Check the Food Label:
4 g of sugar = 1 teaspoon of sugar = 5 mL
8 ounces (oz) = 1 cup = 250 mL
16 oz = 500 mL
32 oz = 1 L
40 oz = 1.2 litres

1 Soft drinks and soda pop. Coke, Pepsi, Mountain Dew, cream soda, ginger ale, Sprite and tonic water. One 12-oz can of soda has a minimum of 7 teaspoons of sugar. Some have 15 teaspoons of sugar. A 16-oz bottle can have up to 20 teaspoons of sugar.

2 Slurpees or iced slushes. The average sized slurpee is 16-oz, with 13 teaspoons of sugar. The super-size 40-oz drink has a half pound (0.2 kg) of sugar. Yikes!

3 Fruit juice. Unsweetened apple juice has even more sugar than regular Coke or Pepsi.

Fruit juice — even without added sugar — is just as fattening as pop.

4 Instant powdered drinks. Iced tea, Tang and Kool-Aid with sugar added have 8 to 11 teaspoons of sugar in 16-oz.

5 Sports drinks. Gatorade and Powerade have sugar, sodium and potassium added. Depending on the brand, the standard sized 16-oz bottle has 9 to 18 teaspoons of sugar added. Of course, the sugar is doubled in a 32-oz bottle.

6 Pre-sweetened coffee-shop coffees and teas. Check online for the nutrients of your favorite specialty coffee or tea. If the drink has 40 g of carbohydrate and 10 g of fat, this means it has 10 teaspoons of sugar and 2 teaspoons of fat.

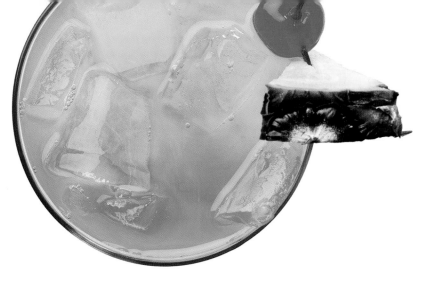

7 **Liquor, wine and beer.** There are 100 to 200 calories in one drink of liquor, wine, beer or cooler. These calories add up into extra pounds of weight on your body.

8 **Commercial smoothies.** When fruits or vegetables are puréed for smoothies, their fiber is chopped so fine that the healthy fiber value is lost. Commercial smoothies have added sugar or honey and are easy to overdrink. Know what you are drinking; check the food label for the number of grams of sugar.

9 **Energy drinks.** Brands like Red Bull, AMP and Monster have added sugar and caffeine. A large (16-oz) has 12 to 14 teaspoons of sugar and as much caffeine as the same sized coffee.

Extra light and low-carb beer has half the calories of regular beer.

10 **Sweetened milk drinks.** Chocolate milk is white milk with 3½ teaspoons of extra sugar in 8-oz. Commercial eggnog and restaurant milkshakes have an excessive amount of sugar added.

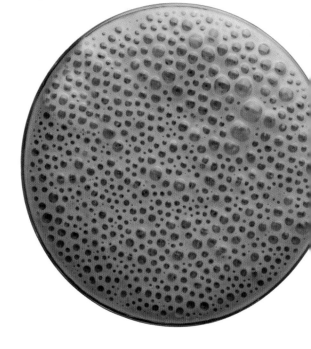

Diabetes-Friendly Beverages

1 **Tap water.** This is your everyday drink. Carry it with you in a reusable water bottle to stay well hydrated.

2 **Flavored tap water.** Add a slice of lemon or lime, berries, sliced cucumber or mint leaves.

On the go? Freeze fruit into ice cubes and add them to your reusable water bottle with reusable straw.

3 **Bottled mineral water, sparkling water or flavored water.** Check the food label to make sure no sugar was added.

4 **Herbal, caffeine-free teas.** Flavorful hot or cold without added sugar.

5 **Coffee and black or green teas.** These drinks have some benefits as antioxidants, especially when you drink them without added sugar, cream or milk.

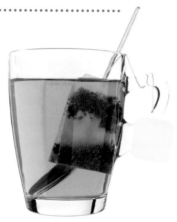

6 **Sugar-free iced tea or lemonade.** Single serving packages of sugar-free iced tea or sugar-free lemonade are convenient. Add to a glass of water and stir, or pour into your water bottle.

7 **Diet drinks.** Sodas and sports drinks with artificial sweeteners are better for your blood sugar than drinking real sugar.

8 **Milk and calcium-rich beverages.** Milk has a natural type of sugar called lactose, which helps absorb calcium into your body. Soy milk is a lactose-free alternative to cow's milk. Other non-dairy milks (such as almond milk) are lower in protein. For best nutritional value, check the label to be sure the milk is unsweetened and has calcium and vitamin D.

9 **Low-salt vegetable juices.** These have natural sugars, but give you healthy plant nutrients with fewer calories and carbs than fruit juice.

10 **Commercial liquid meal replacements.** Diabetes brands have extra fiber, which helps to slow the rise of your blood sugar. If your appetite is poor, one of these small bottles has the calories of a small meal.

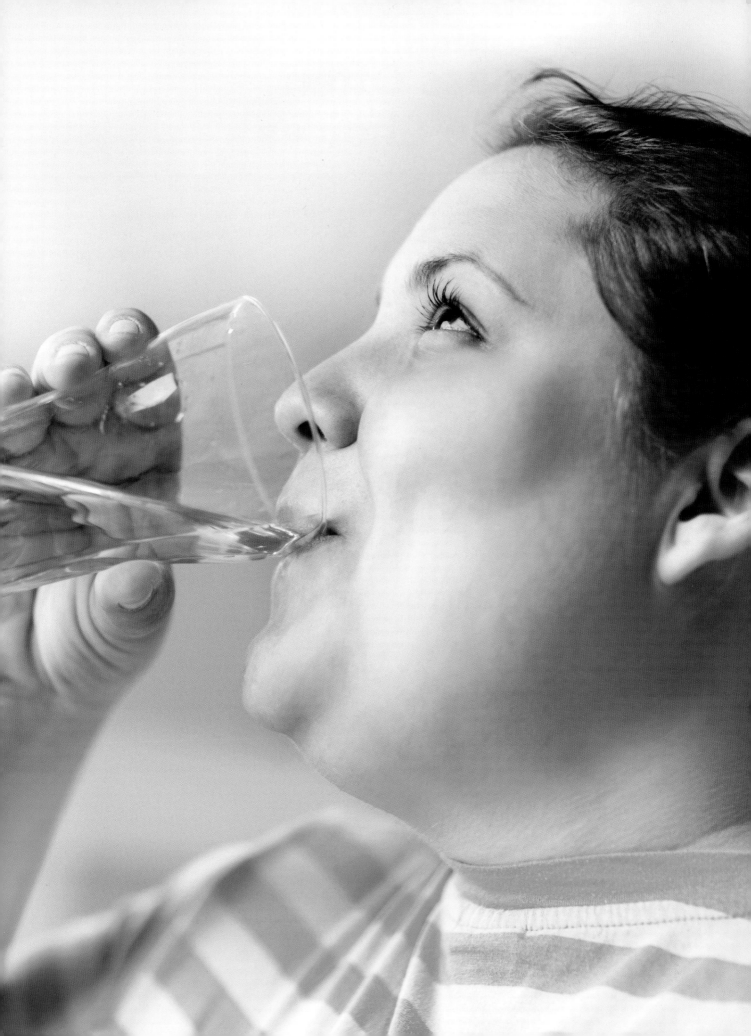

Eat Out Less Often — Make Wise Choices

1 Plan. Decide what you will eat before you go out. Check the restaurant menu online for calories in the main meal, sides and beverages. You will be less likely to over-order.

2 How to manage buffets. Use a smaller plate. Be mindful and choose smaller amounts of food to taste on your first trip, then go back for what you like.

3 Is a salad meal healthier? Not necessarily. Salads are often served with high-fat salad dressing, deep fried chicken and garlic bread on the side. These calories add up quickly.

4 Substitute healthier choices. Try one of these:
- sliced tomatoes instead of hash browns
- diet drink instead of regular
- salad with the dressing on the side
- grilled chicken, not crispy

5 Share desserts. Fancy specialty desserts are delicious and loaded with calories. Feel like cheesecake or chocolate cake? Half a slice is plenty to finish off a meal.

6 Box it up. A large restaurant meal may be enough for two dinners. Take half home and you have dinner for the next day!

7 How to manage potlucks. Bring a healthy choice:
- a fruit plate with Greek yogurt dip
- a vegetable tray with hummus
- sushi or vegetable-filled rice paper spring rolls (or lettuce rolls)

8 How to manage holiday feasting. It's an easy time to overeat — both in restaurants and at family parties. If you're the host, reduce the sugar, salt and fat in your cooking. And at meals, try using a smaller plate.

9 Prepare for a walk. Prepare for a 15-minute or longer walk when you get home from eating out. Have your walking shoes ready by the door. Walking helps your digestion, reduces your blood sugar and you will sleep better that night.

10 Travel and restaurant meals. If you travel for work, choose motel rooms with kitchenettes to prepare smaller meals you like. All-inclusive holiday destinations, resorts and cruises can be rewarding — until you gain five to seven pounds in one week.

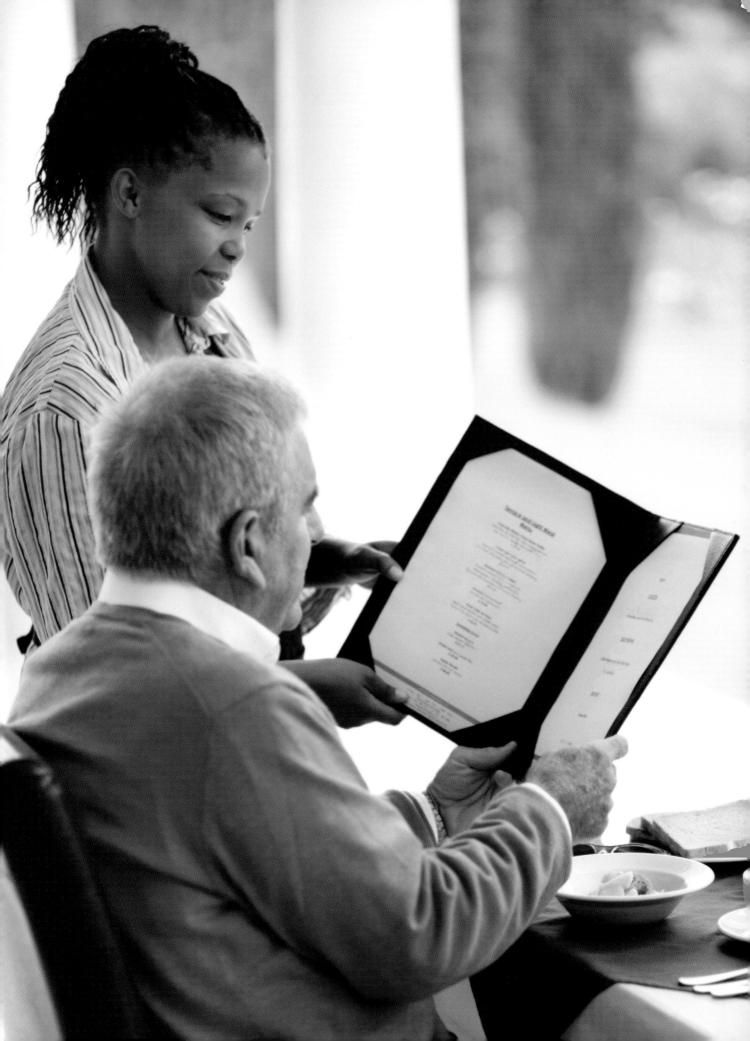

Diabetes Food Questions

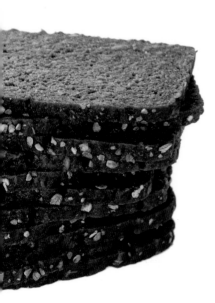

1 Is rye bread better than whole wheat or whole grain bread? These are all good high fiber choices. Whole grain breads with unground grains have the lowest glycemic index. However, always look for bread that is sliced thinly and marked at about 70 calories per slice.

2 Is white bread a forbidden food? No food is forbidden. White bread is low in fiber, so try to combine it with fiber foods like chunky peanut butter.

3 Can I put bread on the table when I'm also serving rice, potatoes or pasta? As a general rule, no.

4 Are artificial sweeteners safe? If they are sold in stores, they have been approved as safe. However, use artificial sweeteners in moderation. A few less common kinds are not approved during pregnancy.

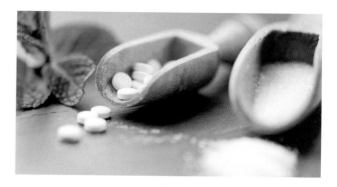

5 What is a good bedtime snack? Try a piece of fruit, a few crackers with cheese or five to 10 almonds. Snack ideas can be found on pages 110–113. If you eat a big snack at night to prevent low blood sugar episodes, you may be taking too much evening insulin — talk to your doctor.

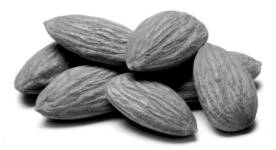

6 Why do I feel hungry? This could be because your blood sugar is raised and you may have insulin resistance. Talk to your doctor about other types of diabetes medication that might reduce your hunger.

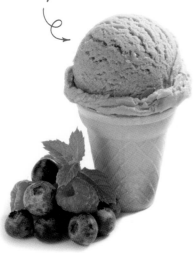

This single scoop ice cream cone has only 150 calories.

7 **What sweets and desserts can I eat?** All desserts will raise your blood sugar. A diabetes dessert should not have more than 250 calories. Restaurant desserts often have 700 or more calories per serving.

8 **What is the difference between starch and sugar?** Both are carbohydrates. Starch is flour, rice, corn, beans, potatoes or pasta. Sugar occurs naturally in milk, fruits and vegetables. White sugar, brown sugar, honey and corn syrup are sugars added to many processed foods.

9 **How do I know how many calories to eat?** If you want to lose weight, here is a guide: 1,200 to 1,800 daily calories for women and 1,500 to 2,200 daily calories for men. Your height, age, physical activity and metabolism all help to determine the number of calories you can eat in a day. To avoid calorie counting, follow the small or large meal plans shown in our diabetes cookbook and our diabetes guide (see page 192).

10 **How many carbs can I eat each day?** As a guide, reduce your daily carbohydrates (carbs) to about half your calories. Higher-fiber carbs such as whole grains, fruits and vegetables are the healthiest. On a 1,200-calorie meal plan, this is about 150 grams of carbs. On a 2,200-calorie meal plan, this would be 275 grams of carbs. The rest of your daily calories can come from proteins and fats. All the recipes in this book show the carbohydrate, protein and fat content for your information.

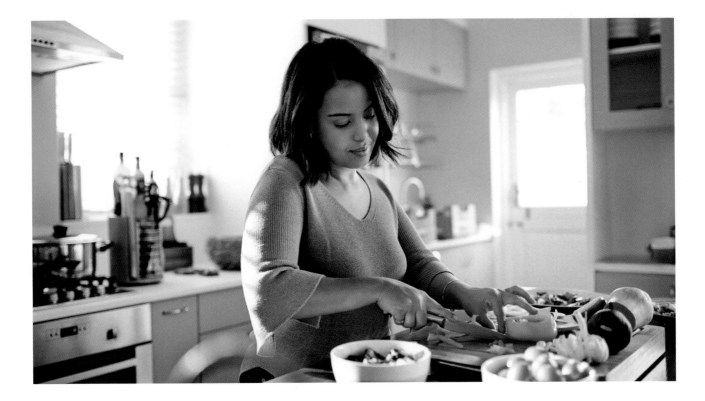

Karen Graham preparing
Chicken Souvlaki (page 99).

Top-Ten Recipes

These diabetes-friendly recipes were created by Karen Graham and tested in her kitchen. Use the 10-day meal plan for a varied diet, and enjoy these dishes with family and friends.

Ten-Day Meal Plan

DAY 1

BREAKFAST
Cold cereal with milk, topped with nuts

SNACK
Fruit

LUNCH
Fish, meat or cheese sandwich (whole-grain bread is a good choice)

Garden Tomato Salad

SNACK
Low-Calorie Vegetable Soup

DINNER
Shake-and-Bake Chicken

Bonnie's Potato Salad

Cauliflower

Mixed vegetables

Fruit

SNACK
Blueberry Oatmeal Muffin

DAY 2

BREAKFAST
English muffin with cheese

SNACK
Chai tea or chilled coffee made with milk

LUNCH
Quinoa Salad or Vermicelli Salad

Hard-boiled egg

SNACK
Sugar-free gelatin

DINNER
Fish Tacos

Poppy Seed Spinach Salad

Brownie

SNACK
Fruit

DAY 3

BREAKFAST
Scrambled egg made with added vegetables

Toast

SNACK
Peanut Butter Oatmeal Cookie

LUNCH
Turkey Noodle Soup

Open-faced toasted tomato and cheese sandwich

SNACK
Pineapple Coleslaw

DINNER
Slow Cooker Pot Roast

Glass of milk

Apple Crumble

SNACK
Popcorn

DAY 4

BREAKFAST
Hot cereal with milk, topped with nuts

SNACK
Fruit

LUNCH
Broccoli Cheese Soup or Potato Leek Soup

Crackers with hummus

Celery sticks

SNACK
2 Slim Bits or a protein bar

DINNER
Vegetarian Chili

Sweet Potato Fries

Avocado Chocolate Pudding

SNACK
Toasted waffle with reduced-sugar pancake syrup

Sugar-free iced tea

DAY 5

BREAKFAST
Toast with peanut butter

Glass of milk

SNACK
Yogurt

LUNCH
Beef Barley Soup or Three Sisters Hamburger Soup

Crackers and cheese

Fruit

SNACK
Carrot sticks

DINNER
Chicken Cobb Salad

Small bun with butter

Slice of Crustless Lemon Meringue Pie

SNACK
Sparkling cranberry water

DAY 6

BREAKFAST
Oatmeal muesli with chia seeds and Greek yogurt

SNACK
Crackers with hummus

LUNCH
Bacon and egg

Toast

Tomatoes

Fruit

SNACK
Small yogurt

DINNER
Pizza

Caesar Salad

Glass of wine or spritzer

Raspberry Cream

SNACK
Herbal tea

DAY 7

BREAKFAST
Tortilla filled with scrambled egg and veggies

Fruit

SNACK
Low-Calorie Vegetable Soup

LUNCH
Sushi rolls with sliced avocado and sliced sweet peppers

SNACK
Slice of Grandma's Zucchini Loaf

DINNER
Barbecue Pork Chops with Grilled Vegetables

Ice Cream Sundae

SNACK
Diet drink

DAY 8

BREAKFAST
Piece of cold pizza

Sliced fruit

SNACK
Piece of cheese

LUNCH
Tuna or salmon sandwich

Carl's Red Cabbage Slaw

SNACK
Sugar-free lemonade

DINNER
Taco Bean Salad

Glass of milk

Fruit with Lime Topping

SNACK
Small bowl of cold cereal with milk

DAY 9

BREAKFAST
Banana Oatmeal Pancake with peanut butter

SNACK
10 pecans or 20 pistachios

LUNCH
Split Pea Soup or Lentil Spinach Soup

Crackers

Raw veggies

SNACK
Fruit

DINNER
Spaghetti Squash Casserole

Everyday Salad

Slice of Ginger Pear Cake

SNACK
Cup of light hot chocolate

DAY 10

BREAKFAST
Avocado Spinach Smoothie

SNACK
Fruit

LUNCH
Peanut butter and banana sandwich

Pumpkin Soup or Fall Tomato Cucumber Soup

SNACK
Diet soft drink

DINNER
Chicken Souvlaki with Tzatziki

Rice or pita

Greek Salad

Fresh fruit sprinkled with cinnamon

SNACK
Glass of tomato juice or tomato-vegetable cocktail juice

Unless otherwise noted, Nutrition Facts in the recipes are based on unsweetened skim or 1% dairy milk, and regular-fat cheese (not "lite" or "reduced fat"). Where there is a choice of ingredients, calculations are based on the first one listed.

TEN TASTY SOUPS

These classic but calorie-light soup recipes can be enjoyed as a snack or as part of a meal. For those that are limiting their salt intake, there is no table salt added to the recipes. Of course, add a little salt to suit your own taste! Freeze extra soup in airtight containers or resealable freezer bags. For best flavor eat homemade soup within four months.

Low-Calorie Vegetable Soup

The great thing about vegetable soup is that you can add the vegetables of your choice. This tasty soup is just under 100 calories per serving. When you have this soup as a start to your meal it helps you cut down on your other meal portions, to help you lose weight. This soup is also a light choice for a midafternoon snack when you might be having a late dinner. **MAKES 8 SERVINGS (EACH 1½ CUPS/375 ML).**

1 tbsp (15 mL) olive oil or vegetable oil

2 cloves garlic, finely chopped

1 small onion, chopped

2 carrots, thinly sliced

1 stalk celery, thinly sliced

2 cups (500 mL) chopped broccoli or green beans

1½ cups (375 mL) shredded green cabbage

28-oz (796 mL) can diced tomatoes with Italian spices, with juice

4 cups (900 mL Tetra Pak) no-salt-added ready-to-use broth (beef, chicken or vegetable)

2½ cups (625 mL) water

2½-oz (70 to 73 g) package instant tomato vegetable soup mix

Salt and pepper to taste

Shredded cheese, optional, to sprinkle on top

1. In a large heavy pot, heat oil over medium heat. Add garlic and onion; sauté for a few minutes until softened. Add carrots, celery, broccoli and cabbage; cook, stirring occasionally, for another few minutes; vegetables will still be slightly firm.

2. Stir in tomatoes with juice, broth, water and soup mix; bring to a boil. Reduce heat to low, cover and simmer, stirring occasionally, for 15 minutes or until vegetables are tender.

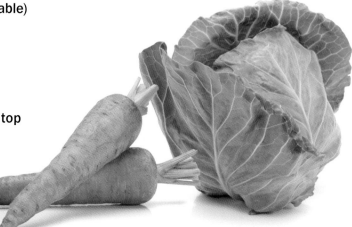

Nutrition Facts PER SERVING

Calories	98	Net Carbs	14 g	Fat, saturated	0 g
Carbohydrate	17 g	Protein	4 g	Cholesterol	0 mg
Fiber	3 g	Fat, total	2 g	Sodium	477 mg

Lentil Spinach Soup

This is such an easy recipe because you don't need to soak the lentils overnight, and it only takes half an hour of cooking. **MAKES 8 SERVINGS (EACH 1½ CUPS/375 ML).**

2 tbsp (30 mL) olive oil or vegetable oil

2 stalks celery, sliced

2 medium carrots, shredded

2 cloves garlic, finely chopped

1 medium onion, chopped

1 cup (250 mL) dried brown or green lentils (whole, not split), rinsed

2 tsp (10 mL) ground cumin

1 tsp (5 mL) ground coriander

½ tsp (2 mL) ground cinnamon

5 cups (1.25 L) water

4 cups (900 mL Tetra Pak) 30%-less-sodium ready-to-use broth (beef, chicken or vegetable)

Juice of 1 lemon (¼ cup/60 mL)

10-oz (300 g) package frozen chopped spinach, thawed

¼ cup (60 mL) chopped fresh cilantro

Salt and pepper to taste

1. In a large heavy pot, heat oil over medium heat. Add celery, carrots, garlic and onion; sauté for 10 minutes or until softened. Add lentils, cumin, coriander and cinnamon; cook, stirring for 2 minutes; this frying helps enhance the flavors of the spices.

2. Stir in water, broth and lemon juice; bring to a boil. Reduce heat to low, cover and simmer for 30 minutes or until lentils are tender.

3. Add spinach and cilantro, stirring until heated through.

This soup is a good source of iron, thanks to the lentils, spinach and cumin.

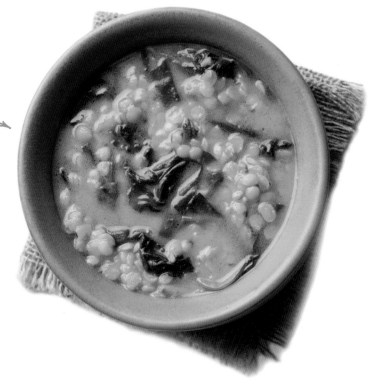

Nutrition Facts PER SERVING

Calories	145	Net Carbs	13 g	Fat, saturated	1 g
Carbohydrate	23 g	Protein	9 g	Cholesterol	0 mg
Fiber	10 g	Fat, total	4 g	Sodium	346 mg

Potato Leek Soup

Leeks are high in antioxidants that keep blood vessels healthy. Leeks have a soluble fiber called inulin, which is especially good for people with diabetes. Leek soup is traditional across Europe. This recipe is superb and still low calorie with the bacon fat included.

MAKES 6 SERVINGS (EACH 1½ CUPS/375 ML).

6 slices bacon, chopped

2 cloves garlic, finely chopped

1 medium onion, chopped

1 leek (white and light green parts only), chopped

3 medium potatoes, peeled and chopped

2 stalks celery, sliced

2 cups (500 mL) fresh, frozen or canned corn kernels

½ tsp (2 mL) pepper

¼ tsp (1 mL) hot pepper flakes or hot pepper sauce

3 cups (750 mL) 2% milk

2 cups (500 mL) no-salt-added ready-to-use broth (beef, chicken or vegetable)

1. In a large heavy pot over medium heat, cook bacon until crisp. Using a slotted spoon, transfer bacon to a plate and set aside.

2. Add garlic, onion and leek to the fat remaining in the pot; sauté for 10 minutes or until softened.

3. Stir in potatoes, celery, corn, pepper, hot pepper flakes, milk and broth; reduce heat to medium and simmer, stirring occasionally, for 20 to 30 minutes or until potatoes are tender. Add the crispy bacon just before serving.

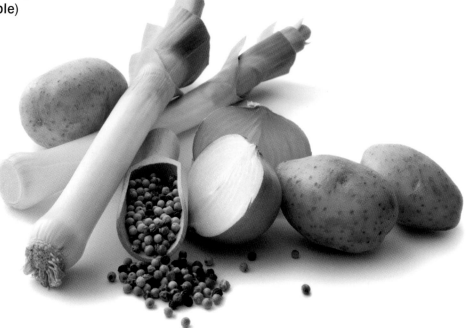

Nutrition Facts PER SERVING

Calories	243	Net Carbs	34 g	Fat, saturated	3 g
Carbohydrate	37 g	Protein	10 g	Cholesterol	20 mg
Fiber	3 g	Fat, total	6 g	Sodium	220 mg

Three Sisters Hamburger Soup

Some Indigenous Peoples of North America traditionally grew corn, climbing beans and squash together. The beans climbed up the corn stalks and the squash leaves shaded the ground, keeping it moist and controlling weeds. This combination of crops came to be known as the "three sisters." **MAKES 10 SERVINGS (EACH 1½ CUPS/375 ML).**

1 lb (500 g) lean ground beef (or wild meat)

4 cloves garlic, finely chopped
   (or 1 tsp/5 mL garlic powder)

1 medium onion, chopped

1 apple, peeled and chopped

4 cups (1 L) diced acorn or butternut squash
   (about 1 small squash)

2 cups (500 mL) fresh, frozen or canned
   corn kernels

2 cups (500 mL) fresh or frozen trimmed
   green bean pieces (½-inch/1 cm pieces)

1 bay leaf

1 tsp (5 mL) dried thyme

1 tsp (5 mL) dried basil

¼ tsp (1 mL) hot pepper flakes or
   a dash of hot pepper sauce

¼ tsp (1 mL) pepper

19-oz (540 mL) can kidney beans,
   drained and rinsed

5½-oz (156 mL) can tomato paste

7 cups (1.75 L) no-salt-added ready-to-use
   broth (beef, chicken or vegetable)

Salt to taste

1. In a large heavy pot over medium heat, cook beef, breaking it up with a spoon. Cook for 15 minutes or until no longer pink. Add garlic and onion; sauté for 5 minutes or until softened.

2. Stir in apple, squash, corn, green beans, bay leaf, thyme, basil, hot pepper flakes, pepper, kidney beans, tomato paste and broth; bring to a boil. Reduce heat to low, cover and simmer, stirring occasionally, for 30 minutes or until vegetables are tender. Discard bay leaf.

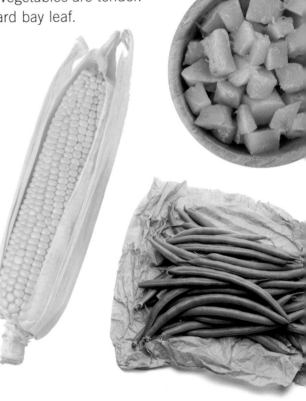

Nutrition Facts PER SERVING

Calories	263	Net Carbs	23 g	Fat, saturated	4 g
Carbohydrate	30 g	Protein	14 g	Cholesterol	32 mg
Fiber	7 g	Fat, total	10 g	Sodium	287 mg

Turkey Noodle Soup

Soups are true comfort food and a great way to get your veggies. This recipe is based on a 15-lb (7 kg) turkey. After you roast a turkey or chicken, boil the bones to make a rich stock, then make the soup the next day. **MAKES 7 SERVINGS (EACH 1½ CUPS/375 ML).**

STOCK WITH MEAT

Bones (meat will still be clinging to some of them) and any extra bits of leftover meat

14 cups (3.5 L) water

SOUP

Stock with meat, from above

3 medium carrots, chopped

2 stalks celery, chopped

1 medium onion, chopped

1 tsp (5 mL) dried dillweed

¼ tsp (1 mL) pepper

2 cups (500 mL) medium or broad egg noodles

Salt to taste

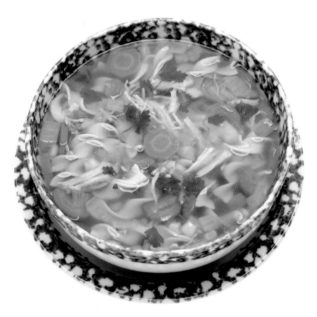

1. To make your stock, cover bones and meat with water in a large heavy pot and bring to a boil over medium-high heat. Reduce heat, cover, and simmer for 2 hours or until all the meat has fallen off the bones.

2. Pour the stock (about 12 cups/3 L) through a sieve set over another large pot. Place on the counter uncovered, to cool.

3. Remove chunks of meat from the sieve and chop or shred them. You should have about 2 cups (500 mL) of meat.

4. Place the meat in an airtight container. Cover the pot of cooled stock. Refrigerate both overnight.

5. The next day, remove and discard fat from the chilled stock. Return the chopped meat to the pot. Add carrots, celery, onion, dill and pepper; bring to a boil over medium-high heat. Reduce heat to low, cover and simmer for 30 minutes.

6. Stir in noodles, increase heat to medium-high and boil for 5 minutes until noodles are cooked but not mushy.

Nutrition Facts PER SERVING

Calories	164	Net Carbs	15 g	Fat, saturated	0 g
Carbohydrate	17 g	Protein	18 g	Cholesterol	41 mg
Fiber	2 g	Fat, total	1 g	Sodium	157 mg

OPTION: For a thicker soup, let it cool slightly, then purée in a blender and reheat before serving.

Pumpkin Soup

This delicious, mild-tasting soup can be made with fresh pumpkin or butternut squash in the fall, or any time of year with canned pumpkin.

MAKES 5 SERVINGS (EACH 1½ CUPS/375 ML).

2 tbsp (30 mL) butter

1 medium onion, chopped

1 medium apple, peeled and chopped

7 cups (1.75 L) cubed pumpkin (about 1 small pumpkin, cut into ½-inch/1 cm pieces)

4 cups (900 mL Tetra Pak) no-salt-added ready-to-use broth (beef, chicken or vegetable)

1 tbsp (15 mL) curry powder

¼ tsp (1 mL) ground cinnamon

2 tbsp (30 mL) all-purpose flour

2 cups (500 mL) skim milk

Salt and pepper to taste

Raw, unshelled pumpkin seeds or sunflower seeds, optional, for topping

1. In a large heavy pot, melt butter over medium heat. Add onion and sauté for 5 minutes or until softened.

2. Stir in apple, pumpkin, broth, curry powder and cinnamon; bring to a boil. Reduce heat and simmer, stirring occasionally, for 45 minutes or until the pumpkin and apple are tender.

3. In a bowl, whisk flour into milk until blended. Stir into soup and simmer. Stir for 5 minutes or until it starts to thicken slightly, and serve.

TIP: In place of the fresh pumpkin, you can use a 28-oz (796 mL) can of 100% pure pumpkin.

Nutrition Facts PER SERVING

Calories	**172**	Net Carbs	**24 g**	Fat, saturated	**3 g**
Carbohydrate	**27 g**	Protein	**7 g**	Cholesterol	**35 mg**
Fiber	**3 g**	Fat, total	**5 g**	Sodium	**128 mg**

Split Pea Soup

This reduced-salt soup is made with fresh pork hocks instead of the traditional salted ham or salted or smoked pork hocks. A pork hock is the knuckle at the end of the leg bone. Pork hocks need extra cooking time to soften the gristle, so cook the stock the night before and make the soup the next day. **MAKES 9 SERVINGS (EACH 1½ CUPS/375 ML).**

STOCK WITH MEAT

2 fresh pork hocks (about 2 lbs/900 g)

14 cups (3.5 L) water

SOUP

Stock with meat, from above

2 cups (500 mL) dried green split peas, rinsed

3 stalks celery with leaves, chopped

2 medium carrots, chopped

2 cloves garlic, minced

1 medium onion, chopped

2 bay leaves

½ tsp (2 mL) dried thyme

¼ tsp (1 mL) hot pepper flakes or a dash of hot pepper sauce

Salt to taste

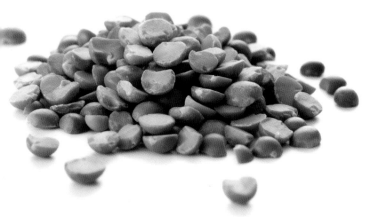

1. To make your stock, put pork hocks and water in a large heavy pot. Bring to a boil then reduce heat to low, cover and simmer for 2 hours or until meat is tender and falling off the bone.

2. Transfer the hocks to a bowl. Let stock and hocks cool.

3. Once the hocks have cooled pull off the skin and fat and remove the meat from the bones. Discard the skin, fat and bones. Chop the meat into small pieces; you should have about 2 cups (500 mL). Place in an airtight container and refrigerate.

4. Once the stock is cool, cover and refrigerate overnight. You will have about 12 cups (3 L).

5. The next day, remove and discard fat from the chilled stock. Add split peas to the stock and bring to a boil over medium to high heat. Reduce heat to low and simmer for 45 minutes, stirring often.

6. Add the reserved meat, celery, carrots, garlic, onion, bay leaves, thyme and hot pepper flakes; return to a boil. Reduce heat, simmer for 15 minutes or until vegetables and split peas are tender. Discard bay leaves.

Nutrition Facts PER SERVING

Calories	167	Net Carbs	16 g	Fat, saturated	0 g
Carbohydrate	26 g	Protein	20 g	Cholesterol	18 mg
Fiber	10 g	Fat, total	1 g	Sodium	120 mg

Fall Tomato Cucumber Soup

Try this savory fall soup made from homegrown garden tomatoes and cucumbers. This puréed soup recipe uses tomato-cucumber juice for the soup base. There will be leftover tomato-cucumber mash that you can freeze and use later in a spaghetti sauce, stew or other soup. **MAKES 7 SERVINGS (EACH 1½ CUPS/375 ML).**

15 medium (or 10 large) tomatoes

2 to 3 large cucumbers, peeled and chopped

2 tbsp (30 mL) butter, margarine or
vegetable oil

4 large cloves garlic, finely chopped

1 medium onion, chopped

2 tbsp (30 mL) all-purpose flour

2 cups (500 mL) 2% milk

2 packages (4.5 g each) reduced-salt
chicken bouillon powder

2 bay leaves

1 tsp (5 mL) dried basil

½ tsp (2 mL) pepper

1. Bring a large heavy pot of water to a boil. Blanch the tomatoes (place them gently in the boiling water for 3 minutes or until skins split). Using a slotted spoon, transfer tomatoes to a bowl and let cool slightly. Peel off skins. Roughly chop tomatoes.

2. Empty pot and return tomatoes to the pot. Add cucumbers to the tomatoes and bring to a simmer over medium heat. Reduce heat and simmer for 30 minutes until softened, stirring occasionally.

3. Let cool slightly, then pour through a sieve set over another large pot and press out the juice with the back of a spoon. This should give about 7 cups (1.75 L) of juice; set aside.

4. Place the tomato and cucumber mash in an airtight container and freeze for later use.

5. In a large, clean pot, melt butter over low to medium heat. Sauté garlic and onion for about 5 minutes or until softened. Stir in flour until blended. Gradually stir in milk, then add the reserved juice, bouillon powder, bay leaves, basil and pepper; bring to a boil, stirring often. Reduce heat and simmer for 15 minutes or until slightly thickened.

6. Remove soup from heat and let cool slightly. Discard bay leaves. Using an immersion blender in the pot, purée soup until smooth, or transfer to a blender in batches to purée. Reheat before serving.

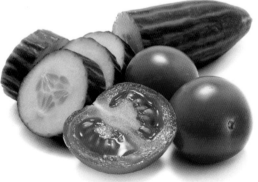

Nutrition Facts PER SERVING

Calories	112	Net Carbs	13 g	Fat, saturated	3 g
Carbohydrate	14 g	Protein	4 g	Cholesterol	15 mg
Fiber	1 g	Fat, total	5 g	Sodium	218 mg

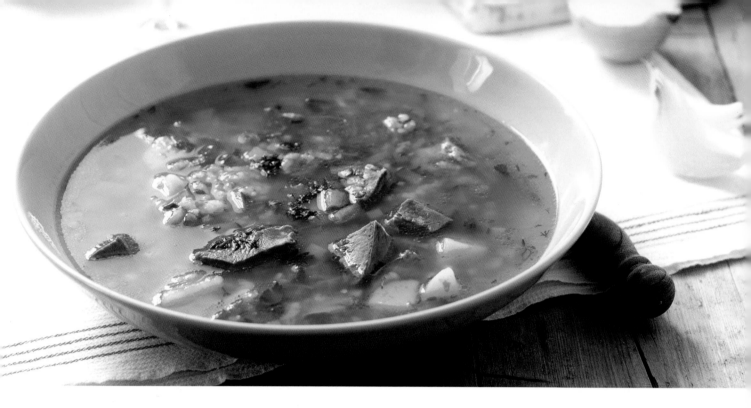

Beef Barley Soup

Make this soup with leftover cooked roast beef or hamburger. This is an easy soup to create, with turnip and pot barley giving unique and flavorful tastes.

MAKES 7 SERVINGS (EACH 1½ CUPS/375 ML).

1 tbsp (15 mL) olive oil or vegetable oil

1 small onion, chopped

2 medium carrots, sliced

2 stalks celery, sliced

3-inch (7.5 cm) turnip, diced

2 cups (500 mL) chopped or shredded cooked beef (or cooked ground beef)

1 cup (250 mL) pot barley

0.9-oz (25 g) brown gravy mix

½ tsp (2 mL) pepper

10 cups (2.5 L) water

Salt to taste

1. In a large heavy pot, heat oil over medium heat. Sauté onion for 5 minutes or until softened.

2. Stir in carrots, celery, turnip, beef, barley, gravy mix, pepper and water; bring to a boil. Reduce heat to low, cover and simmer, stirring occasionally, for about 1 hour or until barley is tender.

Nutrition Facts PER SERVING

Calories	234	Net Carbs	21 g	Fat, saturated	4 g
Carbohydrate	25 g	Protein	10 g	Cholesterol	29 mg
Fiber	4 g	Fat, total	11 g	Sodium	210 mg

Broccoli Cheese Soup

This popular soup is delicious made with broccoli or cauliflower. Leave it chunky to maintain the fiber and for a lower GI. For guests, purée the soup for a special occasion. Make it the day ahead, so you'll have more time on the day your guests arrive.
MAKES 5 SERVINGS (EACH 1½ CUPS/375 ML).

2 tbsp (30 mL) butter

1 medium onion, chopped

1 medium potato, peeled and diced

5 cups (1.25 L) coarsely chopped broccoli

2 cups (500 mL) no-salt-added ready-to-use broth (beef, chicken or vegetable)

3 cups (750 mL) skim milk

½ tsp (2 mL) pepper

1 cup (250 mL) shredded Cheddar cheese

Salt to taste

Additional shredded Cheddar cheese, optional, for topping

1. In a large heavy pot, melt butter over low to medium heat. Sauté onion for 5 minutes or until softened.

2. Stir in potato, broccoli and broth; bring to a boil. Reduce heat to low, cover and simmer for 20 minutes or until vegetables are tender, stirring occasionally.

3. If you are choosing to purée this soup, let it cool slightly. Using an immersion blender in the pot, purée soup until smooth, or transfer to a blender in batches.

4. Stir in milk and pepper and return to a simmer over medium heat. Lastly, stir in cheese until melted.

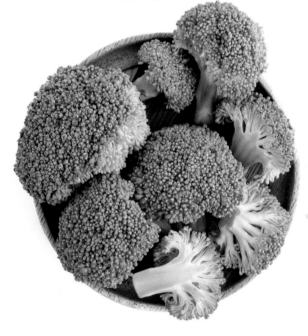

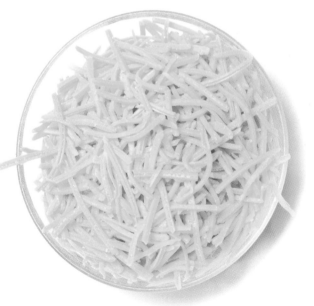

Nutrition Facts PER SERVING

Calories	257	Net Carbs	20 g	Fat, saturated	8 g
Carbohydrate	23 g	Protein	14 g	Cholesterol	39 mg
Fiber	3 g	Fat, total	8 g	Sodium	292 mg

Salads can be adapted to what is fresh and available in the stores or in your garden. Most of the vegetables used in salads are low in calories and high in nutrients; the calories come from the dressing. Side salads can be eaten with any meal or enjoyed as a snack. Add roasted chicken, boiled eggs or cheese to turn any side salad into a meal.

Everyday Salad

This colorful salad with fruit is fast and easy to make. Change the fruit for a new flavor and a new look each time you make it. **MAKES 4 SERVINGS.**

4 cups (1 L) torn salad greens

3 radishes, sliced

2 green onions, sliced

1 large tomato, cut into small wedges

$\frac{1}{2}$ cucumber, peeled and diced

$\frac{1}{2}$ cup (125 mL) fruit (such as blueberries, orange segments, pomegranate seeds or chopped apple or pear)

4 to 6 tbsp (60 to 90 mL) light salad dressing (40 calories or less per tbsp/15 mL)

1. In a large bowl, combine salad greens, radishes, green onions, tomato, cucumber and fruit. Drizzle dressing over top and toss gently to coat.

TIPS: *In place of the green onions, you can use $\frac{1}{4}$ small red onion, sliced into rings.*

If you choose English cucumbers, you won't have to peel them. They have a more tender skin.

Salad greens are easy to grow — and you can pick them every day.

Nutrition Facts PER SERVING

Calories	73	Net Carbs	7 g	Fat, saturated	1 g
Carbohydrate	9 g	Protein	2 g	Cholesterol	0 mg
Fiber	2 g	Fat, total	4 g	Sodium	156 mg

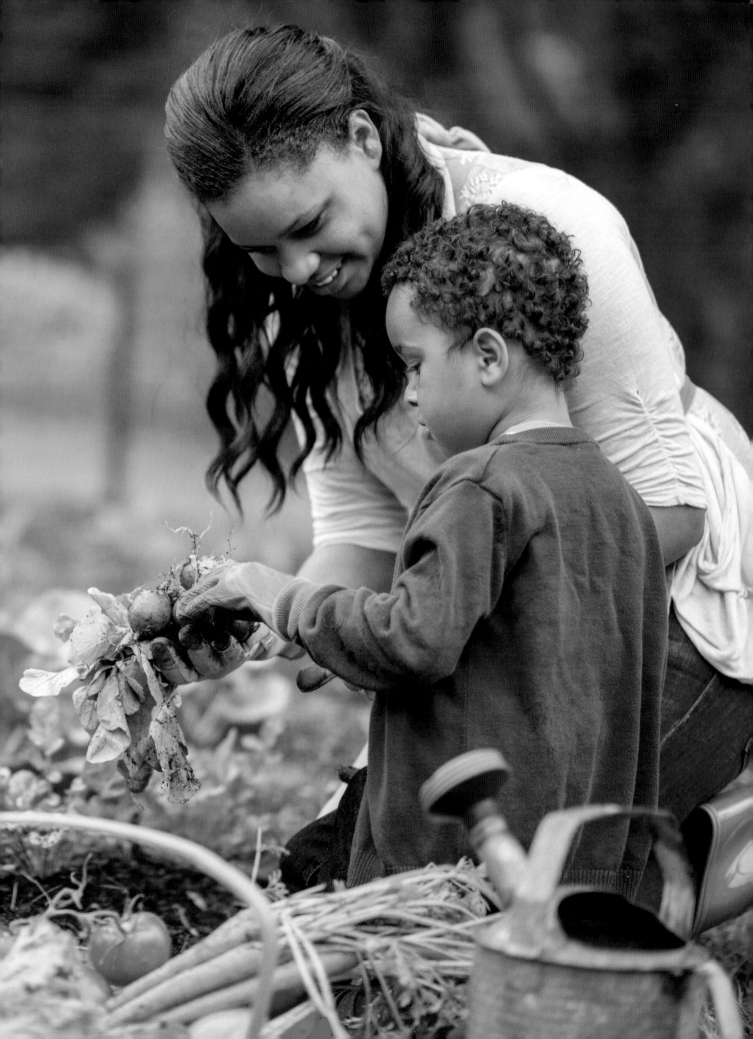

Caesar Salad

Some of the best things in life are simple. This is true for this Caesar salad with just four ingredients. **MAKES 4 SERVINGS.**

4 cups (1 L) torn dark salad greens

4 to 6 tbsp (60 to 90 mL) light Caesar salad dressing (40 calories or less per tbsp/15 mL)

½ cup (125 mL) lightly packed Parmesan cheese, shaved or shredded from a wedge

½ cup (125 mL) croutons

1. Place salad greens in a large bowl, drizzle with dressing and toss gently to coat.

2. Add cheese and croutons.

Nutrition Facts PER SERVING

Calories	113	Net Carbs	7 g	Fat, saturated	2 g
Carbohydrate	8 g	Protein	6 g	Cholesterol	13 mg
Fiber	1 g	Fat, total	6 g	Sodium	287 mg

Greek Salad

This traditional Greek salad is fast and easy to make. It can be enjoyed as a side salad with lamb, chicken or beef souvlaki, or grilled pork or fish. Everything goes well with Greek salad! This recipe was originally developed for our diabetes cookbook. **MAKES 2 SERVINGS.**

2 large tomatoes, cut into wedges

½ medium red onion, sliced

½ green bell pepper, cut into chunks

½ small cucumber, cut into chunks

12 small black olives (or 4 large)

¼ cup (60 mL) feta cheese, crumbled or in small chunks

1 tbsp (15 mL) olive oil

1 tbsp (15 mL) red wine vinegar

1 tsp (5 mL) dried oregano

1. In a large bowl, combine tomatoes, onion, green pepper, cucumber, olives and feta cheese.

2. In a small bowl, whisk together oil, vinegar and oregano. Pour over salad and toss to coat.

Nutrition Facts PER SERVING

Calories	205	Net Carbs	15 g	Fat, saturated	4 g
Carbohydrate	17 g	Protein	5 g	Cholesterol	17 mg
Fiber	2 g	Fat, total	15 g	Sodium	478 mg

Carl's Red Cabbage Slaw

Karen's son developed this recipe while living in Colombia. Lime is a staple ingredient throughout South and Central America and Mexico. It enhances the flavor of so many dishes. **MAKES 5 SERVINGS (EACH 1 CUP/250 ML).**

3 medium carrots, shredded

4 cups (1 L) thinly sliced red cabbage

Juice of 1 lime (2 tbsp/30 mL)

1 tbsp (15 mL) olive oil

1 tbsp (15 mL) soy sauce

1 tbsp (15 mL) pure maple syrup

1 tsp (5 mL) minced or grated gingerroot
  (or ½ tsp/2 mL ground ginger)

Pinch of pepper

Dash of hot pepper sauce, optional

1. In a large bowl, combine carrots and cabbage.

2. In a small bowl, whisk together lime juice, oil, soy sauce, maple syrup, ginger and pepper.

3. Pour dressing over cabbage mixture and toss to coat.

TIP: To prepare the cabbage, cut it in half and place flat side down. With a large knife, cut thin slices, then cut the slices crosswise into bite-size pieces.

Nutrition Facts PER SERVING

Calories	**76**	Net Carbs	**8 g**	Fat, saturated	**0 g**
Carbohydrate	**11 g**	Protein	**4 g**	Cholesterol	**0 mg**
Fiber	**3 g**	Fat, total	**3 g**	Sodium	**229 mg**

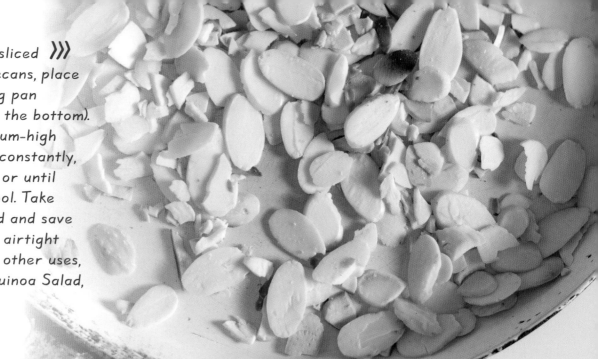

TIP: To toast sliced ⟫⟫⟫ almonds or pecans, place in a dry frying pan (enough to fill the bottom). Toast on medium-high heat, stirring constantly, for 2 minutes or until golden. Let cool. Take what you need and save the rest in an airtight container for other uses, such as the Quinoa Salad, page 87.

Poppy Seed Spinach Salad

This colorful salad of greens and reds is an attractive choice when you have guests for dinner. This recipe also appears in our diabetes cookbook. **MAKES 2 SERVINGS.**

3½ cups (875 mL) fresh spinach, lightly packed

1 medium tomato, cut into small wedges

¼ small red onion, sliced into rings

½ cup (125 mL) sliced strawberries, pomegranate seeds, or seedless orange segments

2 tbsp (30 mL) sliced almonds or pecans, lightly toasted

3 tbsp (45 mL) reduced-fat (light) creamy poppy seed salad dressing (40 calories or less per tbsp/15 mL)

Sprinkle of poppy seeds, optional, for topping

1. In a large bowl, combine spinach, tomato, onion, strawberries and almonds.

2. Drizzle with dressing and toss gently to coat.

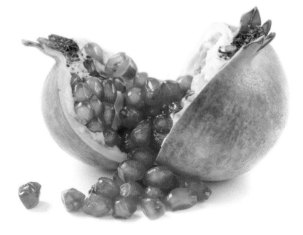

Nutrition Facts PER SERVING

Calories	142	Net Carbs	15 g	Fat, saturated	1 g
Carbohydrate	18 g	Protein	4 g	Cholesterol	0 mg
Fiber	3 g	Fat, total	9 g	Sodium	146 mg

Vermicelli Salad

This salad has visual appeal with the matchstick-thin sliced vegetables and fruit.
MAKES 6 SERVINGS (EACH 1½ CUPS/375 ML).

4 oz (125 g) dry vermicelli rice noodles

Boiling water

2 medium carrots, grated

1 English cucumber (unpeeled), cut into thin matchsticks

1 small apple, pear or mango, cut into thin matchsticks

¼ red onion (or 2 green onions), thinly sliced

½ cup (125 mL) chopped fresh cilantro

½ cup (125 mL) unsalted peanuts, chopped

DRESSING

2 cloves garlic, minced

2 tbsp (30 mL) olive oil

1 tbsp (15 mL) soy sauce or fish sauce

1 tbsp (15 mL) pure maple syrup

1 tbsp (15 mL) white vinegar

¼ tsp (1 mL) hot pepper flakes or a dash of hot pepper sauce

Pinch of salt

1. In a large heatproof bowl or pot, cover vermicelli noodles with boiling water and let stand for 3 minutes or until soft. Rinse under cold water and drain.

2. Place noodles in a large salad bowl. Add carrots, cucumber, apple, onion and cilantro, tossing to combine.

3. **Dressing:** In a small bowl, whisk together garlic, oil, soy sauce, maple syrup, vinegar, hot pepper flakes and salt.

4. Pour dressing over noodle mixture and toss to coat evenly. Sprinkle with peanuts.

Vermicelli are thin rice noodles popular in Vietnamese and other Asian cuisines. Rice noodles are prepared for soups, stir-fries and salads.

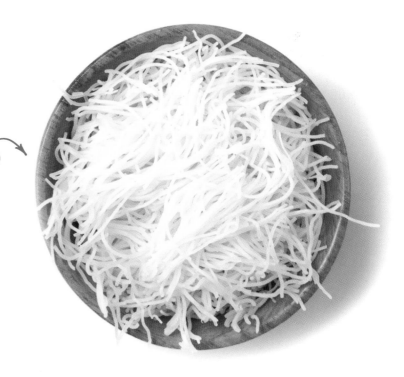

Nutrition Facts PER SERVING

Calories	222	Net Carbs	27 g	Fat, saturated	2 g
Carbohydrate	30 g	Protein	5 g	Cholesterol	0 mg
Fiber	3 g	Fat, total	10 g	Sodium	203 mg

Bonnie's Potato Salad

Karen's neighbor shared this family recipe, which has been influenced over time by different cultures. It has elements of Dutch, German and Canadian Prairie cooking.

MAKES 8 SERVINGS (EACH 1 CUP/250 ML).

4 medium (about 3-inch/7.5 cm round) potatoes (see tip, below), peeled and cut into quarters for boiling

2 large eggs

1 medium carrot, peeled and grated

4 large radishes, ends removed, grated

1 stalk of celery plus leaves, chopped

2 medium green onions or 4 stalks of chives, sliced

1 large dill pickle, chopped

1 small apple, peeled, cored and chopped

1/2 cup (125 mL) light mayonnaise or Original Miracle Whip

1 tbsp (15 mL) prepared mustard

1/4 tsp (1 mL) salt

1/4 tsp (1 mL) pepper

Sprinkle of fresh dill, finely chopped, optional

Sprinkle of paprika, optional

TIP: *Yukon gold or red potatoes hold their shape best for potato salads.*

SAFETY TIP: *Salad recipes that call for mayonnaise or Miracle Whip need to be kept in the fridge or served right away.*

1. Place potatoes and eggs in a saucepan and add enough cold water to cover. Bring to a boil over high heat. Reduce heat and boil gently for 10 minutes. Remove the eggs and cool in cold water. Simmer the potatoes for another 3 minutes or until fork-tender (be sure not to overcook). Drain potatoes and cool in cold water, and cut into 1/2-inch (1 cm) chunks.

2. Peel and chop the eggs.

3. In a large bowl, stir together mayonnaise, mustard, salt and pepper. Add potatoes, eggs, carrot, radishes, celery, green onions, dill pickle and apple. Serve sprinkled with sprigs of dill and paprika, if desired.

Try different flavored mustards available in specialty stores.

Nutrition Facts PER SERVING

Calories	131	Net Carbs	17 g	Fat, saturated	1 g
Carbohydrate	19 g	Protein	3 g	Cholesterol	52 mg
Fiber	2 g	Fat, total	5 g	Sodium	277 mg

Quinoa Salad

Quinoa is a seed from a flowering plant that thrives in high altitudes. It is native to South America and is now being grown in other parts of the world too. Quinoa has a mild flavor and is high in protein, making it a great addition to salads. This dressing has a vibrant taste with a choice of alcohol or non-alcohol flavoring.

MAKES 6 SERVINGS (EACH 1 CUP/250 ML).

1 small (3-inch/7.5 cm) beet

½ cup (125 mL) quinoa, rinsed

⅓ cup (75 mL) sliced almonds, toasted (see page 84)

6 cups (1.5 L) lightly packed greens, such as arugula and spinach

⅓ cup (75 mL) dried cranberries

⅓ cup (75 mL) crumbled feta cheese

WHISKEY DRESSING

½ tsp (2 mL) dry mustard

½ tsp (2 mL) garlic powder

¼ tsp (1 mL) salt

2 tbsp (30 mL) reduced-sugar pancake syrup

1½ tbsp (22 mL) whiskey or bourbon (or 1½ tsp/7 mL vanilla or rum extract)

1½ tbsp (22 mL) apple cider vinegar or any other flavored vinegar

1 tbsp (15 mL) vegetable oil or olive oil

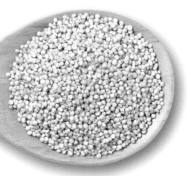

1. Poke several fork holes in the beet and place in a microwave-safe dish with a small amount of water. Microwave on High for 4 minutes. Or boil the beet for 30 minutes until tender.

2. Let the beet cool. Slice off the ends, peel and cut into thin slices. Set aside.

3. Bring 4 cups (1 L) water to a boil. Stir in quinoa, reduce heat and simmer, uncovered, for 12 minutes until quinoa is tender. Drain through a fine-mesh sieve and rinse under cold running water until cool. Drain well and set aside.

4. **Whiskey Dressing:** In a small bowl, whisk together mustard, garlic powder, salt, syrup, whiskey, vinegar and oil.

5. In a large salad bowl, combine quinoa, greens, cranberries and feta. Drizzle with the dressing and toss gently to combine.

6. Divide quinoa salad evenly among six salad bowls and top with sliced beets and toasted almonds.

TIP: This salad becomes a full meal for 4 larger servings when topped with sliced roasted chicken or baked salmon.

Nutrition Facts PER SERVING

Calories	206	Net Carbs	20 g	Fat, saturated	2 g
Carbohydrate	24 g	Protein	6 g	Cholesterol	7 mg
Fiber	4 g	Fat, total	8 g	Sodium	219 mg

Pineapple Coleslaw

The flavor of this Pineapple Coleslaw will remind you of summer any time of the year. Select pre-cut packaged cabbage coleslaw mix from the grocery store to speed up prep time; this is also a great crunchy snack. **MAKES 5 SERVINGS (EACH 1 CUP/250 ML).**

1 stalk celery, finely chopped

4 cups (1 L) coleslaw mix

1 cup (250 mL) crushed pineapple, drained (see tip)

¼ cup (60 mL) reduced-fat (light) coleslaw dressing

1. In a large bowl, combine celery, coleslaw mix and pineapple.

2. Drizzle with dressing and toss to coat evenly.

TIP: A 14-oz (400 mL) can of crushed pineapple will give you the 1 cup (250 mL) drained pineapple, with enough left over to add to a fruit salad.

Nutrition Facts PER SERVING

Calories	58	Net Carbs	8 g	Fat, saturated	0 g
Carbohydrate	10 g	Protein	2 g	Cholesterol	4 mg
Fiber	2 g	Fat, total	1 g	Sodium	153 mg

Garden Tomato Salad

In this salad, the tomato gets the spotlight it deserves. For best flavor, select fresh tomatoes from your garden or from the local farmers' market. **MAKES 2 SERVINGS.**

1 large tomato, cut into wedges (or 20 cherry tomatoes, halved)

1 tbsp (15 mL) coarsely chopped fresh basil

1 clove garlic, minced

1 tbsp (15 mL) olive oil

1½ tsp (7 mL) balsamic or flavored vinegar such as apple cider vinegar

Pepper

1. In a bowl, combine tomatoes and basil to taste.

2. In a small bowl, whisk together garlic, oil, vinegar and pepper to taste.

3. Drizzle over tomato mixture and toss gently to coat.

Nutrition Facts PER SERVING

Calories	83	Net Carbs	4 g	Fat, saturated	1 g
Carbohydrate	5 g	Protein	1 g	Cholesterol	0 mg
Fiber	1 g	Fat, total	7 g	Sodium	5 mg

TEN HEARTY DINNERS

These are comfort meals, where family of all ages can learn to cook these wholesome foods and share quality time together. Or, if you're cooking for one, stock your freezer with soul-satisfying leftovers for busy days. Divide portions on your plate: fill a quarter of your plate with the meat or other protein choice; fill another quarter of your plate with rice or other grains, pasta, corn or potatoes; and fill the remaining half of your plate with vegetables.

Chicken Cobb Salad Dinner

This layered, classic American salad is colorful and has a perfect blend of flavors and textures. Fry the bacon and boil the eggs ahead of time and use up extra cooked chicken from another meal. You can quickly prepare the rest of the salad for a complete dinner meal. **MAKES 2 SERVINGS.**

4 cups (1 L) torn lettuce (bite-size pieces)

1 avocado, sliced

1/3 cup (75 mL) crumbled blue cheese
  or shredded Cheddar cheese

4 oz (125 grams) cooked chicken, sliced
  (or 1 cup/250 mL cooked chicken, chopped)

1 tomato, cut into wedges

4 slices crisply cooked bacon, chopped

2 large eggs, hard-boiled, chilled and sliced

1/4 cup (60 mL) coleslaw dressing
  (or your favorite dressing)

1. Divide lettuce between two large dinner plates. On top of the lettuce, arrange in rows the avocado, cheese, chicken, tomato, bacon and egg.

2. Serve with dressing on the side or drizzle it on top.

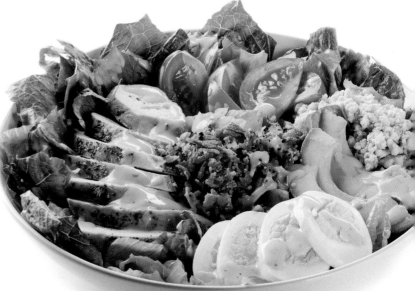

Nutrition Facts PER SERVING

Calories	454	Net Carbs	11 g	Fat, saturated	8 g
Carbohydrate	17 g	Protein	39 g	Cholesterol	274 mg
Fiber	6 g	Fat, total	27 g	Sodium	832 mg

Fish Tacos

The secret to this fabulous Mexican recipe is the tangy sauce. **MAKES 1 SERVING.**

¼ cup (60 mL) finely shredded cabbage
  or lettuce

Several thin slices red bell pepper

Several thin slices red onion

2 tbsp (30 mL) Taco Sauce (recipe at right)

3 oz (90 g) skinless white fish

Salt and pepper to taste

1 tsp (5 mL) vegetable oil

Two 5-inch (12.5 cm) whole-grain flour tortillas
  (or one 10-inch/25 cm tortilla)

¼ small avocado, sliced

1 tbsp (15 mL) chopped fresh cilantro

Wedge of lime on the side, optional

1. In a bowl, toss together cabbage, red pepper, red onion and Taco Sauce. Refrigerate until ready to use.

2. Season fish with salt and pepper. In a skillet, heat oil over medium-high heat. Add fish and cook, turning once, for a few minutes per side or until fish is opaque and flakes easily when tested with a fork.

3. If desired, warm tortilla(s) for 10 seconds per side in a dry frying pan over medium to hot heat.

4. Arrange cabbage mixture down the center of tortilla(s). Place fish on top. Top with avocado and cilantro. If using small tortillas, serve them open; for a large tortilla, roll it up and cut it in half.

Taco Sauce
MAKES ABOUT ½ CUP (125 ML)

You will have some of this sauce left over. It is also tasty as the dressing on the Taco Bean Salad (page 97) or as a condiment on a hamburger.

1 clove garlic, finely chopped
1 tbsp (15 mL) finely chopped chives
  or green onions
½ tsp (2 mL) each: chili powder, paprika,
  ground cumin, ground coriander
  and salt
½ cup (125 mL) light mayonnaise or
  7% sour cream
1 tbsp (15 mL) freshly squeezed lime
  juice

1. Combine all ingredients in a blender. Process the sauce until smooth.

2. Cover and refrigerate for up to 5 days.

Nutrition Facts
PER 2 TBSP (30 ML):
66 Calories, **2 g** Net Carbs,
1 g Protein, **6 g** Fat and
460 mg Sodium.

TIP: Instead of the chili powder, you can use 1 chipotle pepper in adobo sauce.

Nutrition Facts PER FISH TACO WITH TACO SAUCE

Calories	437	Net Carbs	31 g	Fat, saturated	3 g
Carbohydrate	38 g	Protein	27 g	Cholesterol	54 mg
Fiber	7 g	Fat, total	21 g	Sodium	853 mg

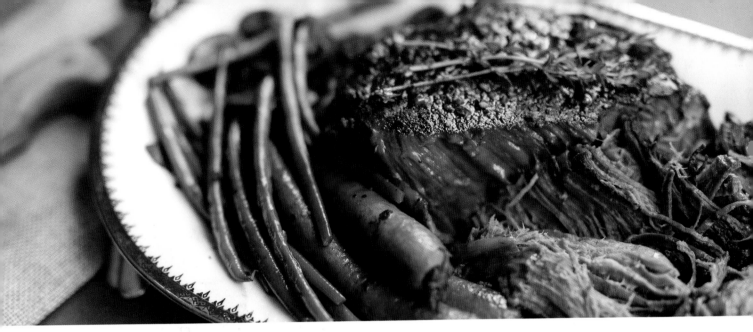

Slow Cooker Pot Roast

Slow cooking turns a tough, lower cost meat into this succulent and fork-tender meal. This recipe holds all the goodness and rich flavor of the meat and vegetables in the sauce. If you don't have a slow cooker, bake the meal in a covered roasting pan in a 325°F (160°C) oven for 4 hours or until meat is tender. **MAKES 10 SERVINGS (EACH 1½ CUPS/375 ML).**

4-lb (2 kg) boneless beef blade roast (or rump or pot roast), trimmed of excess fat

2 medium onions, chopped in chunks

3 small potatoes, chopped in chunks

3 medium carrots, chopped in chunks, or 6 whole baby carrots

2 cups (500 mL) chopped vegetables (such as celery, mushrooms or bell peppers) and/or green or yellow beans, trimmed

10-oz (284 mL) can condensed cream soup, any choice; low sodium options available

½ cup (125 mL) no-salt-added ready-to-use vegetable or beef broth or water

½ cup (125 mL) dry red wine or light beer

Half of a 1-oz (28 g) package dry onion soup mix

1 tsp (5 mL) dried thyme or rosemary, or several fresh sprigs

¼ tsp (1 mL) pepper

1. Place roast in a 4 to 6 quart slow cooker and arrange onions, potatoes, carrots and vegetables around it.

2. In a small bowl, whisk together soup, broth, wine, onion soup mix, thyme and pepper. Pour over roast and vegetables.

3. Cover and cook on High for 4 hours or on Low for 8 hours, until meat is tender.

4. Refrigerate leftovers in a sealed container for up to 3 days or freeze for up to 6 months.

Nutrition Facts PER SERVING

Calories	**527**	Net Carbs	**15 g**	Fat, saturated	**7 g**
Carbohydrate	**17 g**	Protein	**63 g**	Cholesterol	**204 mg**
Fiber	**2 g**	Fat, total	**20 g**	Sodium	**483 mg**

Vegetarian Chili with Sweet Potato Fries

This is a great meal for Meatless Monday, or any day of the week. If there are any leftovers of this chili, it tastes even better the next day. **MAKES 6 SERVINGS (EACH 1½ CUPS/375 ML).**

2 tbsp (30 mL) butter, margarine or vegetable oil

2 cloves garlic, finely chopped

1 medium onion, chopped

1½ tsp (7 mL) chili powder

1½ tsp (7 mL) dried oregano

1 tsp (5 mL) ground cumin

1 bell pepper (any color), cut into chunks

1 small zucchini or eggplant, cut into chunks

1½ cups (375 mL) diced butternut or acorn squash or pumpkin

28-oz (796 mL) can diced tomatoes, with juice

19-oz (540 mL) can mixed beans, drained and rinsed (2 cups/500 mL)

½ cup (125 mL) frozen, canned or fresh corn kernels

Salt and pepper to taste

¼ cup (60 mL) chopped fresh cilantro, optional

1. In a large pot, melt butter over medium heat. Add garlic and onion; sauté for 5 minutes until softened. Add chili powder, oregano and cumin; sauté for 1 minute. Add bell pepper, zucchini and squash; sauté for 2 minutes.

2. Stir in tomatoes with juice, beans and corn; bring to a boil. Reduce heat to low, cover and simmer, stirring occasionally, for about 1½ hours or until vegetables are tender.

3. Serve with sweet potato fries.

Sweet Potato Fries
MAKES 3 SERVINGS
(EACH 18 3-INCH FRIES)

1 6-inch (15 cm)/10½-oz (300 g) sweet potato, with skin

1 tbsp (15 mL) olive oil or vegetable oil

1 tsp (5 mL) ground cumin

1. Wash, dry and slice sweet potato into about 54 sticks.

2. Toss with vegetable oil. Sprinkle with ground cumin.

3. Arrange in a single layer on a rimmed baking sheet, either oiled or lined with parchment paper.

4. Bake in a 450°F (225°C) oven for 20 minutes, turning once.

Nutrition Facts
PER SERVING (18 FRIES)
130 Calories, **18 g** Net Carbs, **2 g** Protein, **5 g** Fat and **57 mg** Sodium.

Nutrition Facts PER SERVING OF VEGETARIAN CHILI

Calories	203	Net Carbs	28 g	Fat, saturated	3 g
Carbohydrate	34 g	Protein	8 g	Cholesterol	10 mg
Fiber	6 g	Fat, total	5 g	Sodium	431 mg

Shake-and-Bake Chicken

The chicken takes minutes to prepare before cooking. This homemade coating has less salt than a store-bought package and is just as delicious every time. **MAKES 4 SERVINGS.**

8 chicken drumsticks (2 lbs/0.92 kg), skin removed

¼ cup (60 mL) Low-Salt Shake-and-Bake Coating (recipe at right)

1. Preheat oven to 375°F (190°C).

2. Place coating in a clean plastic bag or plastic container with a lid. Add drumsticks one at a time, and shake to coat. Place on a greased, rimmed baking sheet. Discard any excess coating.

3. Bake for 45 minutes until no pink shows when you cut into a chicken piece.

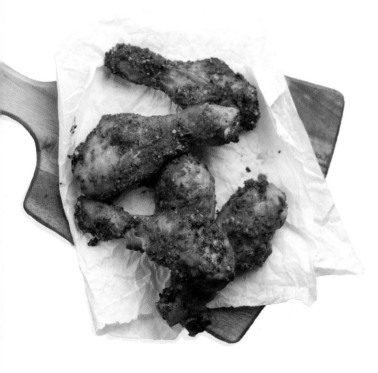

Low-Salt Shake-and-Bake Coating

MAKES ABOUT 1 CUP (250 ML)

½ cup (125 mL) fine dry bread crumbs

¼ cup (60 mL) all-purpose flour

2 tbsp (30 mL) cornstarch

2 tsp (10 mL) paprika

1 tsp (5 mL) each: chili powder, garlic powder, onion powder, ground thyme, ground sage and ground rosemary

½ tsp (2 mL) pepper

¼ tsp (1 mL) ground nutmeg

1 package (about 5 g) low-sodium chicken bouillon powder

1. In a container, glass jar or sealable plastic bag, combine bread crumbs, flour, cornstarch, paprika, chili powder, garlic powder, onion powder, thyme, sage, rosemary, pepper, nutmeg and bouillon powder. Cover or seal and shake to blend.

2. This makes four times enough coating for this chicken recipe. Store the rest in your cupboard if you plan to use it up within the next month. Otherwise, store it in your freezer for up to a year.

Nutrition Facts: PER 1 TBSP (15 ML) COATING (FOR 2 DRUMSTICKS): **26** Calories, **5 g** Net Carbs, **1 g** Protein, **0 g** Fat and **35 mg** Sodium.

Nutrition Facts PER 2 COOKED CHICKEN DRUMSTICKS WITH COATING

Calories	280	Net Carbs	5 g	Fat, saturated	3 g
Carbohydrate	5 g	Protein	39 g	Cholesterol	140 mg
Fiber	0 g	Fat, total	10 g	Sodium	177 mg

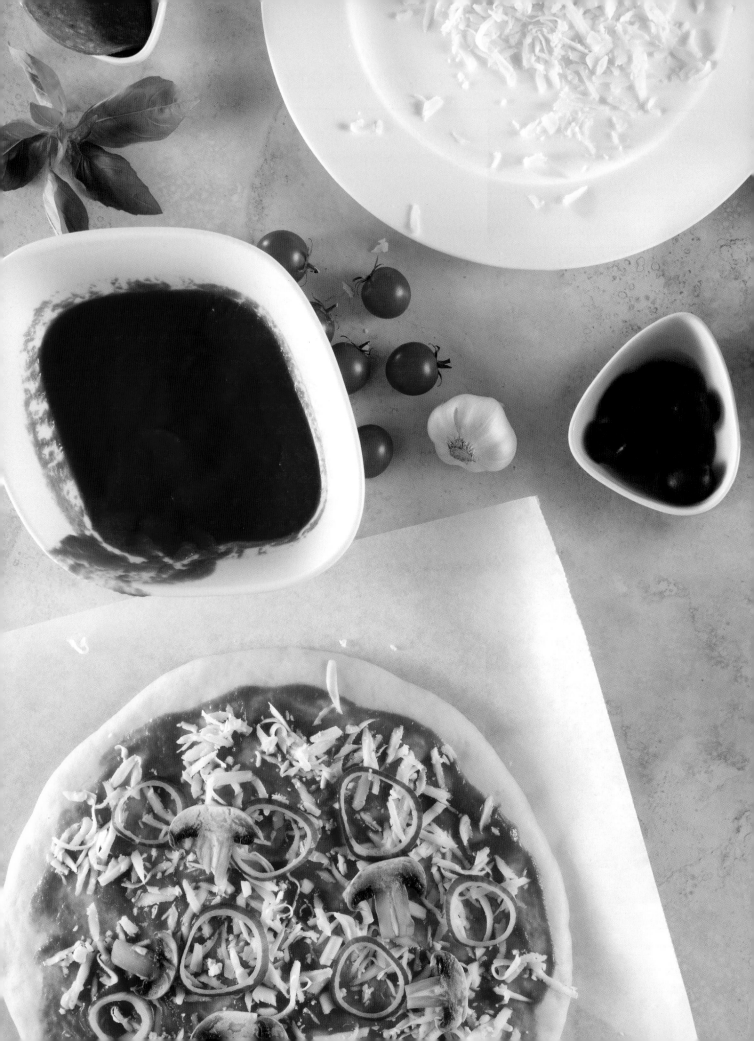

Pizza

Make this quick homemade pizza tonight! Using a ready-made pizza crust and your favorite toppings, you'll have dinner on the table in 15 minutes. Thin-crust pizza shells are generally half the calories and carbs per portion. They can be half the cost too, since you can get two-for-one in the package. **MAKES ONE 12-INCH (30 CM) PIZZA (6 SLICES).**

3 tbsp (45 mL) water

1 tbsp (15 mL) vegetable oil

1 medium onion, thinly sliced

12-inch (30 cm) ready-made thin- or thick-crust pizza shell

½ cup (125 mL) pizza sauce

1 to 2 cups (250 to 500 mL) thinly sliced vegetables (such as bell peppers, mushrooms or tomatoes)

1 cup (250 mL) shredded mozzarella cheese

Other Topping Ideas

➤ **Low-sodium protein:** Sliced roasted chicken or cooked hamburger, fresh salmon or shrimp

➤ **Higher-sodium meats:** Sliced pepperoni, ham, sausage, bacon or smoked salmon

➤ **Fruits:** Pineapple pieces (for Hawaiian pizza), thin slices of pear or fresh figs

➤ **Olives:** Black or green

➤ **Herbs:** Dried or fresh basil or oregano

➤ **Baby arugula:** tossed with balsamic vinegar and olive oil; put this topping on after it comes out of the oven

1. Preheat oven according to pizza shell package directions, usually 450°F (230°C).

2. In a skillet, heat water and oil over medium heat. Add onion and sauté for 5 minutes until softened. The water reduces the amount of oil needed.

3. Place pizza shell on a baking sheet and spread pizza sauce evenly over top, leaving a ½-inch (1 cm) border. Top with sautéed onion. Add vegetables. Sprinkle cheese evenly over top.

4. Bake according to package directions, usually 8 minutes, or until crust is crisp and cheese is melted and starting to brown.

TIP: You can use a pasta sauce instead of the pizza sauce, if you have one on hand. But it may be thinner. So use a sieve to drain off any excess liquid.

OPTION: For an even easier meal, buy a ready-made cheese pizza and top it with vegetables and sautéed onion before baking.

Nutrition Facts PER SLICE OF THIN CRUST PIZZA (THICK CRUST PIZZA)

Calories	176 (251)	Net Carbs	17 g (29 g)	Fat, saturated	4 g (4 g)
Carbohydrate	18 g (31 g)	Protein	6 g (8 g)	Cholesterol	10 mg (10 mg)
Fiber	1 g (2 g)	Fat, total	9 g (10 g)	Sodium	296 mg (408 mg)

Barbecued Pork Chops with Grilled Vegetables

The best thing about barbecuing is the cooking outdoors! Start your vegetables first as they take longer to cook than the meat. **MAKES 4 SERVINGS.**

¼ cup (60 mL) water

¼ cup (60 mL) soy sauce

1 tbsp (15 mL) vegetable oil or olive oil

1 tsp (5 mL) no-salt-added garlic and herb seasoning

⅛ tsp (0.5 mL) pepper

4 pork chops without bone (1.5 lbs/0.670 kg), trimmed of fat

1. In a small bowl, whisk together marinade ingredients: water, soy sauce, oil, seasoning and pepper. (Makes about ½ cup/125 mL, enough for 4 pork chops.)

2. Place pork chops in a shallow casserole dish and pour marinade over top. Cover and refrigerate for several hours or overnight.

3. Oil the barbecue grill and preheat to medium-high heat.

4. Remove pork chops from marinade; discard the marinade. Grill pork chops for 10 minutes (5 minutes per side) or to desired doneness. Cooking time will depend on the thickness of the pork chops and the heat of your barbecue.

TIP: If you don't have a barbecue, place your food on a rimmed baking sheet and grill in your oven to desired doneness.

Grilled Vegetables
SERVES 2

1 medium potato, skin on, chopped into small hash brown size

4 cups of your favorite vegetables, cut into chunks (try red onion, bell pepper, zucchini, yellow summer squash, mushrooms, eggplant, asparagus or Brussels sprouts)

2 tbsp (30 mL) vegetable oil or olive oil

2 tsp (10 mL) dried oregano

1 tsp (5 mL) no-salt-added garlic and herb seasoning

1. Place potato and vegetables in a large bowl.

2. Drizzle with vegetable oil and sprinkle with oregano and seasoning.

3. Transfer to a non-stick perforated grilling skillet and place on the barbecue at medium-high heat. Cook for about 30 minutes, or to desired doneness, stirring occasionally for consistent cooking.

Nutrition Facts PER SERVING
239 Calories, 22 g Net Carbs, 4 g Protein, 15 g Fat and 14 mg Sodium.

Nutrition Facts PER PORK CHOP

Calories	272	Net Carbs	0 g	Fat, saturated	3 g
Carbohydrate	0 g	Protein	41 g	Cholesterol	104 mg
Fiber	0 g	Fat, total	11 g	Sodium	525 mg

Taco Bean Salad Dinner

Try a vegetarian meat substitute made from soy protein, such as Original Veggie Ground Round. Or, if using ground beef, cook it in a heavy pan at medium heat, breaking it up with a spoon, for 15 minutes until cooked through, then drain off the fat. **MAKES 4 SERVINGS.**

312 g pouch ready-to-eat meat substitute such as Original Veggie Ground Round or ½ lb (250 g) lean ground beef, pre-cooked

19-oz (540 mL) can black beans, drained and rinsed

12-oz (341 mL) can corn kernels, drained

2 tsp (10 mL) chili powder

1 tsp (5 mL) ground cumin

1 tsp (5 mL) dried oregano

1 tsp (5 mL) paprika

1 tsp (5 mL) garlic powder

½ tsp (2 mL) pepper

6 cups (1.5 L) torn lettuce or other leafy greens (about ½ head)

2 large tomatoes, chopped or cut into wedges

1 green bell pepper, sliced

⅓ cup (75 mL) light creamy salad dressing, any choice

1 cup (250 mL) shredded Cheddar cheese

50 g (20 chips) tortilla chips

1. **If using ready-to-eat meat substitute,** put it in a frying pan, and add the beans, corn, chili powder, cumin, oregano, paprika, garlic powder and pepper. Stir frequently at medium heat for 5 minutes to heat through. **If using ground beef,** add the above ingredients to the pan where the beef has been pre-cooked. Stir at medium heat for 5 minutes, until everything is heated through.

2. In a large bowl, toss together lettuce, tomatoes and green pepper. Add the meat substitute or meat mixture and salad dressing. Stir gently.

3. Divide salad among four wide serving bowls or plates. Top with cheese and tortilla chips.

Nutrition Facts PER SERVING MADE WITH VEGGIE GROUND (GROUND BEEF)

Calories	493 (552)	Net Carbs	39 g (36 g)	Fat, saturated	6 g (11 g)
Carbohydrate	52 g (46 g)	Protein	31 g (28 g)	Cholesterol	30 mg (70 mg)
Fiber	13 g (10 g)	Fat, total	20 g (30 g)	Sodium	1257 mg (911 mg)

Spaghetti Squash Casserole

This casserole is baked until golden brown and is absolutely yummy. Strands of spaghetti squash look like spaghetti, but have much less carbohydrate than real spaghetti. This meal can be made vegetarian by swapping the ground beef with 468 g (1½ pouches) of ready-to-eat meat substitute made from soy protein, such as Original Veggie Ground Round.
MAKES 6 SERVINGS.

2½-lb (1.25 kg) spaghetti squash (about 7 inches/18 cm long)

¾ lb (375 g) lean ground beef

1½ cups (375 mL) tomato basil sauce

1½ cups (375 mL) 1% or 2% cottage cheese

¼ cup (60 mL) freshly grated Parmesan cheese

1 tsp (5 mL) dried parsley

¼ tsp pepper

1 large egg

1½ cups (375 mL) shredded mozzarella cheese

TIP: Choose a jarred or canned tomato basil sauce that has about 50 calories per ¹/₂ cup (125 mL).

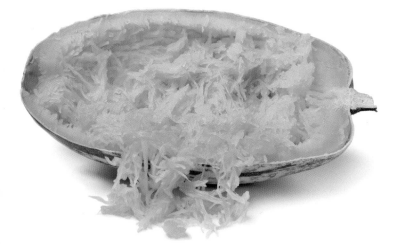

1. Preheat oven to 375°F (190°C). Grease a glass baking dish 13- by 9-inch (33 by 23 cm) or 10-inch (25 cm) square.

2. Using a sharp knife, poke holes in the squash at least ½ inch (1 cm) deep. Microwave squash on High for 4 minutes. Turn squash over and microwave for another 4 minutes or until tender in the center. Let stand in the microwave for 10 minutes to cool slightly.

3. Cut squash in half and scoop out and discard seeds. Using a fork, scrape out flesh in long strands. Set aside.

4. In a large frying pan over medium heat, cook beef, breaking it up with a spoon, for 15 minutes until no pink remains. Drain off the fat. Stir in tomato basil sauce, reduce heat and simmer for 10 minutes.

5. In a large bowl, combine cottage cheese, Parmesan, parsley, pepper and egg.

6. Spread half the squash in prepared baking dish. Top with beef mixture, then cheese mixture, then the remaining squash. Sprinkle mozzarella evenly over top.

7. Bake for 20 minutes or until cheese is bubbling.

Nutrition Facts PER SERVING

Calories	356	Net Carbs	11 g	Fat, saturated	14 g
Carbohydrate	13 g	Protein	28 g	Cholesterol	97 mg
Fiber	2 g	Fat, total	22 g	Sodium	700 mg

Chicken Souvlaki with Tzatziki

Souvlaki is a popular Greek food made with chunks of meat or vegetables grilled on a skewer. This marinade is deliciously flavored with garlic, oregano, rosemary and lemon. Serve with Tzatziki and Greek Salad (see page 82). **MAKES 8 SKEWERS.**

4 cloves garlic, finely chopped

1 tbsp (15 mL) dried oregano

1 tsp (5 mL) dried rosemary

1/2 tsp (2 mL) salt

1/2 tsp (2 mL) pepper

2 tbsp (30 mL) olive oil

Juice of 1 large lemon (2 tbsp/30 mL)

1 1/2 lbs (750 g) boneless skinless chicken breasts, cut into 1-inch (2.5 cm) pieces

1. In a large bowl, combine marinade ingredients: garlic, oregano, rosemary, salt, pepper, oil and lemon juice. Add chicken pieces and toss in marinade until well coated. Marinade overnight or several hours before grilling.

2. Soak skewers in water for 30 minutes to prevent them from burning.

3. Preheat barbecue grill to medium.

4. Remove chicken from marinade and discard marinade. Thread 5 pieces of chicken onto each skewer. Grill for 15 minutes until chicken is no longer pink inside. Turn skewers occasionally to cook meat on all sides.

TIP: If you don't have a barbecue, you can place the skewers on a rimmed baking sheet and grill in your oven to desired doneness.

Tzatziki

MAKES ABOUT 3 CUPS (750 ML)

This is a great way to eat plain yogurt — so thick and creamy made with shredded cucumbers. It's the perfect dipping sauce for your chicken souvlaki.

1 medium English cucumber, with about half the peel removed, grated

1 clove of garlic, finely chopped or minced

1 tsp (5 mL) granulated sugar

1/2 tsp (2 mL) dried dillweed

1/8 tsp (0.5 mL) salt

2 cups (500 mL) 0% to 2% plain Greek yogurt

1 tsp (5 mL) freshly squeezed lemon juice

1. Using your hands, in small batches, squeeze the liquid from the shredded cucumber. Place in a medium bowl and gently stir in garlic, sugar, dill, salt, yogurt and lemon juice.

2. Serve immediately or cover and refrigerate for up to three days.

Nutrition Facts PER 1/4 CUP (60 ML): 28 Calories, **3 g** Net Carbs, **4 g** Protein, **0 g** Fat and **41 mg** Sodium.

Nutrition Facts PER SKEWER OF CHICKEN SOUVLAKI

Calories	105	Net Carbs	1 g	Fat, saturated	1 g
Carbohydrate	1 g	Protein	18 g	Cholesterol	49 mg
Fiber	0 g	Fat, total	3 g	Sodium	134 mg

Apple Crumble

Crumbles can be made year-round but are especially great in the fall, when fruit comes into season. Serve with a spoonful of yogurt or a piece of cheese. **MAKES 9 SERVINGS (EACH ½ CUP/125 ML).**

5 medium apples, peeled and sliced

½ cup (125 mL) quick cooking oats

½ cup (125 mL) packed brown sugar

¼ cup (60 mL) whole wheat flour

¼ cup (60 mL) all-purpose flour

1 tsp (5 mL) ground cinnamon

¼ cup (60 mL) butter, softened, or margarine

1. Preheat oven to 375°F (190°C).

2. Place apples in an ungreased 8-inch (20 cm) square baking dish.

3. In a bowl, combine oats, brown sugar, whole wheat flour, all-purpose flour, cinnamon and butter. Using a fork or your fingers, mix together until crumbly. Sprinkle evenly over apples.

4. Bake for 45 minutes or until apples are soft. Let sit for 10 minutes and serve warm.

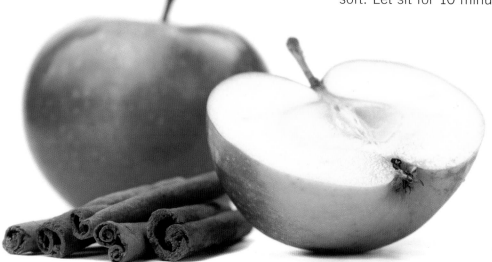

Nutrition Facts PER SERVING

Calories	167	Net Carbs	28 g	Fat, saturated	3 g
Carbohydrate	30 g	Protein	2 g	Cholesterol	13 mg
Fiber	2 g	Fat, total	6 g	Sodium	41 mg

Fruit with Lime Topping

This is such an easy dessert, and can be enjoyed as a healthy snack too. Lime is a small fruit but has impressive benefits. It is rich in vitamin C, an antioxidant that helps keep gums and skin healthy. **MAKES 6 SERVINGS (EACH 1 CUP/250 ML).**

1 cup (250 mL) light (5%) sour cream or plain 0% to 2% Greek yogurt

2 tbsp (30 mL) liquid honey or pure maple syrup

Grated zest of 1 lime

1 tbsp (15 mL) freshly squeezed lime juice

4½ cups (1.1 L) berries or any combination of sliced fresh or canned fruit

1. In a bowl, whisk together sour cream, honey, lime zest and lime juice.

2. Divide fruit among 6 serving bowls and dollop with lime topping.

Nutrition Facts PER SERVING

Calories	81	Net Carbs	12 g	Fat, saturated	1 g
Carbohydrate	13 g	Protein	2 g	Cholesterol	7 mg
Fiber	1 g	Fat, total	2 g	Sodium	64 mg

Avocado Chocolate Pudding

This dessert has a smooth texture and lots of chocolate flavor. It's nutritious too because the avocado is a great source of healthy monounsaturated fats. **MAKES 4 SERVINGS (EACH ½ CUP/125 ML).**

½ cup (125 mL) skim milk or non-dairy milk

1 oz (30 g) semisweet chocolate (or 2 tbsp/ 30 mL semisweet chocolate chips)

2 small ripe avocados, peeled and pitted

3 tbsp (45 mL) unsweetened cocoa powder

¼ cup (60 mL) reduced-sugar pancake syrup

½ tsp (2 mL) vanilla

1. Place milk and chocolate in a small microwave-safe bowl and microwave on High for 20 seconds until melted; stir until smooth.

2. Use an immersion blender in the bowl or transfer to a blender. Combine milk and melted chocolate, avocados, cocoa, syrup and vanilla and blend for 10 seconds until smooth.

Nutrition Facts PER SERVING

Calories	170	Net Carbs	13 g	Fat, saturated	2 g
Carbohydrate	18 g	Protein	3 g	Cholesterol	1 mg
Fiber	5 g	Fat, total	10 g	Sodium	48 mg

Ice Cream Sundae

To keep this sundae as a light dessert, the chocolate sauce is made by you, mixed and heated up in the microwave. All ingredients can be personalized for a great sundae any time of the year. **MAKES 1 SUNDAE.**

½ tsp (2 mL) unsweetened cocoa powder

½ tsp (2 mL) granulated sugar

1 tbsp (15 mL) 2% or whole milk

1 pineapple ring (or 2 tbsp/30 mL crushed or cubed pineapple, drained)

½ cup (125 mL) ice cream

1 tbsp (15 mL) sliced almonds, toasted (see page 84)

1 maraschino cherry, optional

1. **Chocolate sauce:** In a small microwave-safe bowl, combine cocoa powder, sugar and milk. Microwave on High for 20 seconds. Stir well.

2. Place the pineapple in a dessert dish and top with ice cream.

3. Drizzle chocolate sauce over ice cream and sprinkle with almonds. Top with maraschino cherry, if using.

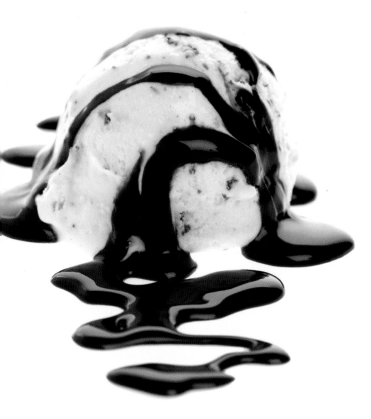

Variations

Pineapple can be replaced with fresh sliced strawberries or banana.

Almonds can be replaced with peanuts, pecans or walnuts.

Cherry on top can be replaced with a few raspberries or blueberries.

Nutrition Facts PER SERVING

Calories	245	Net Carbs	27 g	Fat, saturated	6 g
Carbohydrate	29 g	Protein	6 g	Cholesterol	35 mg
Fiber	2 g	Fat, total	12 g	Sodium	77 mg

Raspberry Cream

This dessert has just three ingredients. Make it in a large glass bowl or 6 individual dessert dishes. This raspberry dessert needs 1½ hours to set and chill, plus another 1 hour to chill before serving. **MAKES 6 SERVINGS (EACH 1¼ CUP/300 ML).**

2 cups (500 mL) frozen raspberries, thawed and drained, at room temperature

1 cup (250 mL) evaporated milk (from a can that was shaken well, before being opened; also see tip, below)

⅓-oz (10 g) package no-sugar-added gelatin powder, such as JELL-O, raspberry or strawberry flavor

1. Place raspberries in dessert bowl or divide between 6 dessert dishes.

2. Pour evaporated milk into a blender, cover and place in the refrigerator to chill.

3. Prepare gelatin according to package directions and refrigerate for 1½ hours until thickened and slightly jiggly but not yet fully set.

4. Blend evaporated milk on high speed for 30 seconds until foamy; it will double in size.

5. Add the thickened gelatin and blend for 10 seconds until smooth.

6. Pour gelatin mixture over raspberries. Cover and chill for another 1 hour before serving (see tip, below).

TIPS: Check the label, and don't buy part-skim (2%) or nonfat (skim) evaporated milk. These variations don't whip up as well. Buy full-fat evaporated milk.

For best quality, note: If the dessert sits for several hours, or overnight, the cream will partially separate.

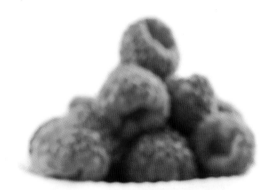

Fresh raspberries can be used in place of frozen.

Nutrition Facts PER SERVING

Calories	80	Net Carbs	7 g	Fat, saturated	1 g
Carbohydrate	9 g	Protein	4 g	Cholesterol	7 mg
Fiber	2 g	Fat, total	3 g	Sodium	128 mg

Brownies

These melt-in-your-mouth brownies are made with a secret ingredient, lentils. These brownies don't need icing; serve with fresh or thawed frozen berries or sliced fruit.
MAKES 15 BROWNIES.

1 cup (250 mL) all-purpose flour

¾ cup (175 mL) unsweetened cocoa powder

⅔ cup (150 mL) granulated sugar

1 tsp (5 mL) baking soda

½ tsp (2 mL) salt

3 large eggs

¾ cup (175 mL) drained rinsed canned lentils (about half a 19-oz/540 mL can)

⅔ cup (150 mL) semisweet chocolate chips

⅔ cup (150 mL) chopped walnuts

½ cup (125 mL) unsweetened applesauce

¼ cup (60 mL) skim milk

1 tsp (5 mL) vanilla

1. Preheat oven to 350°F (180°C). Grease a 13- by 9-inch (33 by 23 cm) metal baking pan.

2. In a large bowl, combine flour, cocoa, sugar, baking soda and salt. Stir well to remove any lumps. Using a wooden spoon, stir in eggs, lentils, chocolate chips, walnuts, applesauce, milk and vanilla until well blended. Use a spatula to scrape the batter into the greased pan and smooth the top of the batter.

3. Bake for 20 minutes or until a tester inserted in the center comes out clean. Cool in the pan.

TIP: Refrigerate or freeze the leftover lentils to use in a soup or stew.

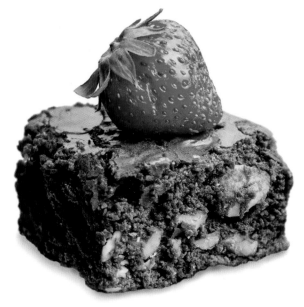

Nutrition Facts PER SERVING

Calories	197	Net Carbs	26 g	Fat, saturated	3 g
Carbohydrate	29 g	Protein	5 g	Cholesterol	37 mg
Fiber	3 g	Fat, total	8 g	Sodium	217 mg

Ginger Pear Cake

You can use fresh pears or apples, or canned pears, to make this fruity cake. It's nice served with a spoonful of vanilla yogurt, and it makes a nice breakfast too! **MAKES 8 SERVINGS.**

½ cup (125 mL) granulated sugar

1 large egg

2 tbsp (30 mL) softened butter or margarine

1 tbsp (15 mL) corn syrup

1 cup (250 mL) all-purpose flour

2 tsp (10 mL) ground ginger

1 tsp (5 mL) cream of tartar

½ tsp (2 mL) baking soda

Pinch of salt

½ cup (125 mL) skim milk

2 pears or apples, peeled and sliced (or 2 canned pears, drained and sliced)

1. Preheat oven to 350°F (180°C). Grease an 8-inch (20 cm) square glass baking dish.

2. In a medium bowl, using a wooden spoon, beat sugar, egg, butter and corn syrup until smooth. Stir in flour, ginger, cream of tartar, baking soda and salt until combined. The mixture will be crumbly. Add milk and stir until batter is smooth.

3. Arrange pears in prepared dish. Gently spread cake mixture over the pears, and smooth the top of the batter.

4. Bake for 30 minutes until knife inserted in the cake comes out clean. Cool in the baking dish.

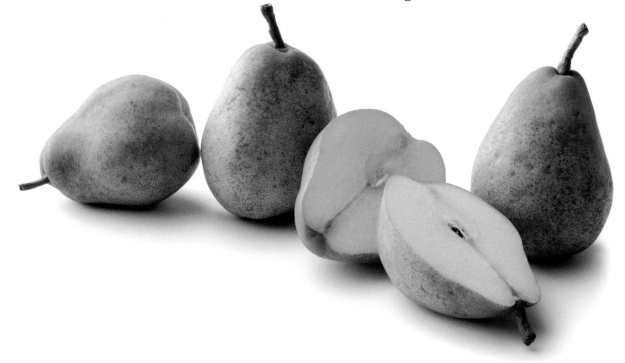

Nutrition Facts PER SERVING

Calories	172	Net Carbs	31 g	Fat, saturated	2 g
Carbohydrate	32 g	Protein	3 g	Cholesterol	35 mg
Fiber	1 g	Fat, total	4 g	Sodium	157 mg

Peanut Butter Oatmeal Cookies

Traditional recipes for peanut butter cookies rely on lots of sugar and fat for their classic flavor. These cookies have rice flour as their essential secret ingredient. Rice flour allows you to use less sugar and fat and still create a soft, flavorful cookie. **MAKES 24 COOKIES.**

½ cup (125 mL) rice flour

¼ cup (60 mL) all-purpose flour

¼ tsp (1 mL) baking soda

¼ tsp (1 mL) salt

½ cup (125 mL) quick cooking oats

¼ cup (60 mL) granulated sugar

2 tbsp (30 mL) butter, softened

1 large egg

½ cup (125 mL) peanut butter

½ tsp (2 mL) vanilla

1. Preheat oven to 375°F (190°C).

2. In a small bowl, sift together rice flour, all-purpose flour, baking soda and salt. Stir in the oats.

3. In a medium bowl, using a wooden spoon, beat sugar and butter until creamy. Beat in egg, peanut butter and vanilla until smooth. Stir in flour mixture until just combined. Don't overmix.

4. Using your hands, form dough into small balls about 1 inch (2.5 cm) in diameter. Place on a greased baking sheet, spacing them about 1 inch apart. Press each ball with the tines of a fork.

5. Bake for 20 minutes or until lightly browned. Immediately remove from baking sheet and transfer to a wire rack to cool.

6. Cookies can be stored in a container on the counter, or can be frozen.

Nutrition Facts PER 2 COOKIES

Calories	138	Net Carbs	13 g	Fat, saturated	2 g
Carbohydrate	14 g	Protein	4 g	Cholesterol	23 mg
Fiber	1 g	Fat, total	8 g	Sodium	75 mg

Grandma's Zucchini Loaf

Grandma's zucchini loaf turns out right every time. The oats and walnuts have extra nutritional value, which is a delight in a dessert. When zucchinis are abundant in the garden, all the neighbors get a loaf too! **MAKES 12 SLICES.**

1½ cups (375 mL) all-purpose flour

⅔ cup (150 mL) quick cooking oats, divided

½ cup (125 mL) chopped walnuts

½ cup (125 mL) granulated sugar

½ tsp (2 mL) salt

½ tsp (2 mL) baking soda

¼ tsp (1 mL) baking powder

½ tsp (2 mL) ground cinnamon

⅛ tsp (0.5 mL) ground nutmeg

2 large eggs

¼ cup (60 mL) vegetable oil

2 tsp (10 mL) vanilla

1¾ cups (425 mL) lightly packed grated zucchini (about 1 medium zucchini)

2 tbsp (30 mL) packed brown sugar

1. Preheat oven to 350°F (180°C). Grease an 8½- by 4½-inch (21 by 11 cm) loaf pan or line it with parchment paper.

2. In a medium bowl, combine flour, ½ cup (125 mL) oats, walnuts, sugar, salt, baking soda, baking powder, cinnamon and nutmeg.

3. In a large bowl, whisk together eggs, oil and vanilla. Stir in zucchini. Add flour mixture in three additions, stirring just until moistened.

4. Spread batter in prepared pan. In a small bowl, combine brown sugar and the remaining oats; sprinkle evenly over the batter.

5. Bake for 1 hour until a tester inserted in the center comes out clean. Immediately remove from the pan and transfer to a wire rack to cool.

Nutrition Facts PER SLICE

Calories	197	Net Carbs	25 g	Fat, saturated	1 g
Carbohydrate	26 g	Protein	4 g	Cholesterol	31 mg
Fiber	1 g	Fat, total	9 g	Sodium	177 mg

Crustless Lemon Meringue Pie

No doubt about it, lemon meringue pie is a sweet treat. This recipe has no crust and so, only half the calories. So put away your guilt and enjoy! Make the pie four hours before you want to serve it, to allow time for it to cool and set. **CUT INTO 8 SERVINGS.**

MERINGUE

3 large egg whites

$\frac{1}{4}$ tsp (1 mL) cream of tartar

$\frac{1}{2}$ tsp (2 mL) vanilla

3 tbsp (45 mL) granulated sugar

FILLING

3 large egg yolks

1 tsp (5 mL) grated lemon zest

$\frac{1}{4}$ cup (60 mL) freshly squeezed lemon juice

2 tbsp (30 mL) cold water

7$\frac{1}{2}$-oz (212 g) package lemon pie-filling and dessert mix

2 cups (500 mL) hot water

TIPS: When separating the eggs, be sure no yolk spills into the egg whites or they won't beat properly.

Refrigerate any leftover pie, covered loosely. After a day or two some of the meringue will separate and become a bit watery.

The nutrient analysis is based on Dr. Oetker Shirriff Original Lemon Pie. If you use a different brand, the ingredients may vary. Use the directions shown here, not those on the box.

1. Preheat oven to 425°F (220°C).

2. In a glass or metal mixing bowl, let egg whites stand at room temperature for 15 minutes.

3. To make your meringue, add cream of tartar and vanilla to the egg whites. Using an electric mixer, beat on high speed until foamy. Gradually beat in sugar until soft peaks form. Set aside.

4. To make your filling, whisk together egg yolks, lemon zest, lemon juice, cold water and pie-filling mix in a medium-size heavy saucepan. Gradually whisk in hot water. Gently whisk constantly over medium-high heat. When bubbles first break the surface, start timing the boil and stir for 30 seconds. Remove from heat.

5. Let the filling cool for 5 minutes, gently whisking twice. It will continue to thicken as it cools.

6. Pour filling into an ungreased 9-inch (23 cm) glass pie plate. While filling is still hot, top with meringue, spreading to the edges.

7. Bake for 4 minutes until meringue is golden. Let cool on a wire rack for 2 hours, then refrigerate until chilled and set, which can take another 2 hours. This pie needs to be cold, so that it will be firm enough to cut into pieces to serve.

Nutrition Facts PER SERVING

Calories	155	Net Carbs	31 g	Fat, saturated	1 g
Carbohydrate	31 g	Protein	2 g	Cholesterol	70 mg
Fiber	0 g	Fat, total	2 g	Sodium	102 mg

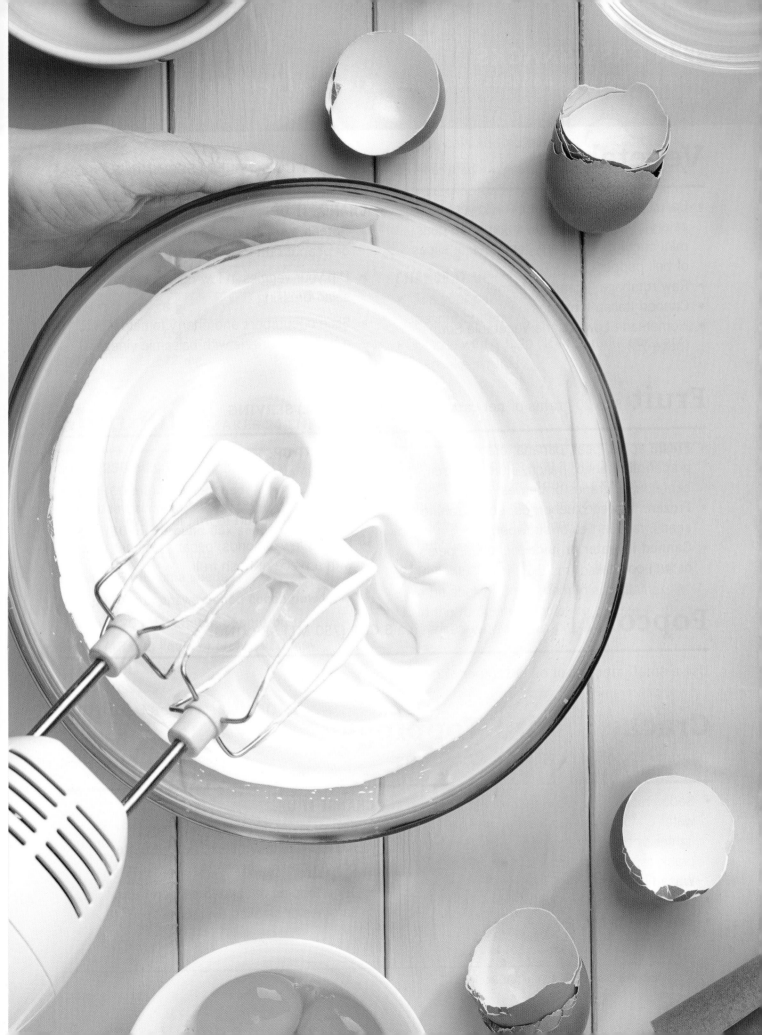

Avocado Spinach Smoothie MAKES 1 SERVING.

¼ small avocado

½ cup (125 mL) raw spinach

1 tsp (5 mL) chia seeds

⅓ cup (75 mL) skim milk

⅓ cup (75 mL) plain yogurt

1 tsp (5 mL) freshly squeezed lemon juice

1. In a blender, combine avocado, spinach, chia seeds, milk, yogurt and lemon juice; blend until smooth. Serve immediately.

You can double the amount of spinach in the smoothie, if you want.

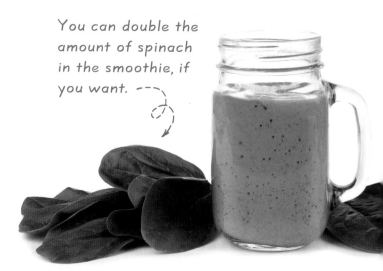

Nutrition Facts

Calories	126
Net Carbs	11 g
Protein	8 g
Fat	5 g
Sodium	103 mg

Cereal 20 grams of net carbs in a 1 CUP (250 ML) SERVING.

- Top your cereal with milk.

TIP: See pages 56–57 for tips on cereal choices.

CHANGE IT UP:

➤ Use lightly sweetened or plain yogurt instead of milk.

➤ Add a pinch of ground cinnamon, nutmeg or cardamom.

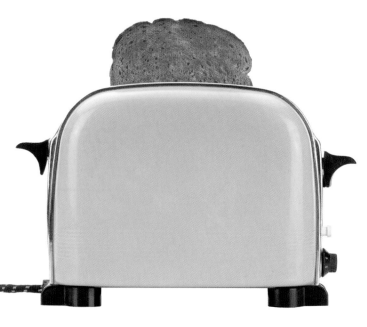

Piece of Toast

15 to 20 grams of net carbs in a **70-CALORIE SLICE OF BREAD, PLUS TOPPING.**

- A slice of toast (such as whole grain, rye or sourdough) with butter or margarine.

CHANGE IT UP:

➤ Spread unbuttered toast with a topping such as peanut butter or another nut butter, honey or jam.

Blueberry Oatmeal Muffins MAKES 12 MUFFINS.

1¼ cups (300 mL) all-purpose flour

½ cup (125 mL) quick cooking oats

½ cup (125 mL) granulated sugar

2 tsp (10 mL) baking powder

½ tsp (2 mL) salt

1 large egg

¾ cup (175 mL) skim milk

¼ cup (60 mL) vegetable oil

1 tsp (5 mL) vanilla

1 cup (250 mL) frozen or fresh blueberries

1 tbsp (15 mL) all-purpose flour

Nutrition Facts

Calories	149
Net Carbs	22 g
Protein	3 g
Fat	5 g
Sodium	122 mg

TIP: *Store-bought and coffee shop muffins typically have 300 to 500 calories — always check the labels and nutrient information, if available, online or at the shop.*

1. Preheat oven to 400°F (200°C). Grease a 12-cup muffin pan.

2. In a large bowl, combine 1¼ cups (300 mL) flour, oats, sugar, baking powder and salt.

3. In a medium bowl, whisk together egg, milk, oil and vanilla until smooth. Pour into flour mixture and stir just to moisten (batter will be lumpy).

4. In a small bowl, mix blueberries with 1 tbsp (15 mL) flour to coat. Fold into batter.

5. Spoon batter into prepared muffin cups, dividing evenly.

6. Bake for 25 minutes or until tops spring back when lightly touched. Immediately remove from pan and transfer to a wire rack to cool.

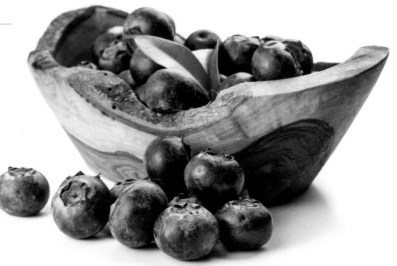

LOOKING FOR MORE SNACK IDEAS?
There are over 200 other snacks in our Health & Wellness series (see page 192); in these books, snacks are grouped into low-calorie small, medium and large.

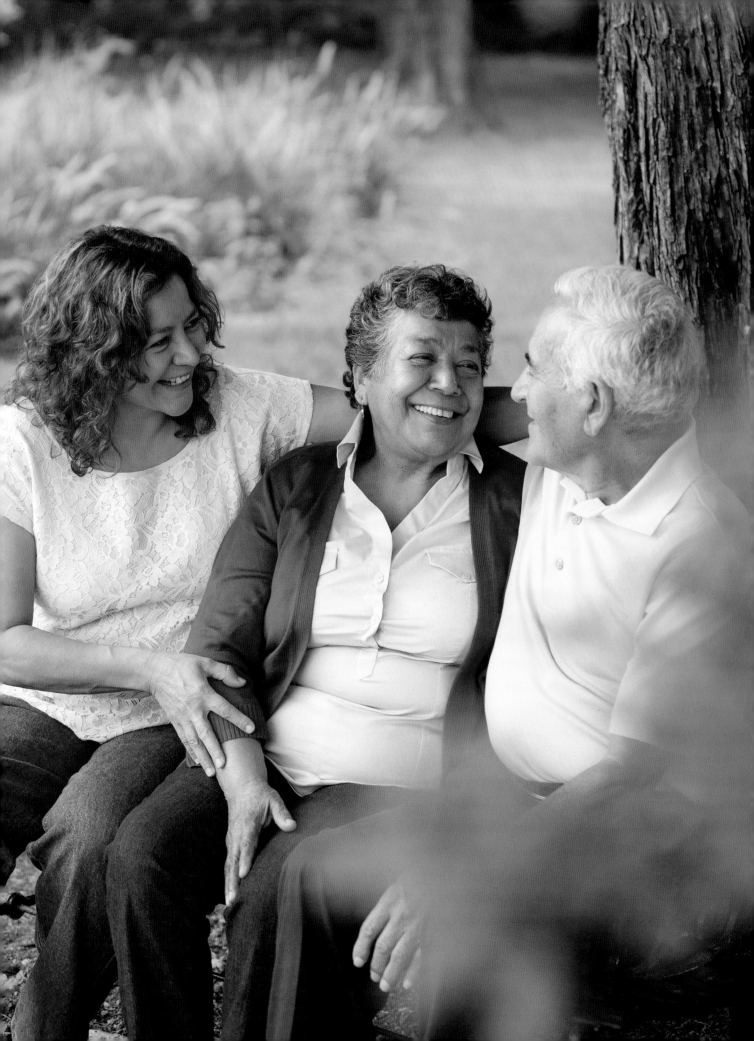

Care for the Whole You

Feeling Overwhelmed with Diabetes

1 Feeling overwhelmed is stressful. Stress raises your blood sugar. Your feelings of stress may be physical feelings of pain, or emotional anger, or mental stresses such as anxiety or depression. When you identify what is stressing you, then you can start working on reducing that stress.

2 Diabetes is a whole body and mind disease. Talk with your doctor. Doctors know that your physical health is connected to your mental health. Your doctor may suggest a short-term sick leave from work or a mental health assessment for short- or long-term counseling. Know who to call if you should need urgent help.

3 New lifestyle. There is a lot to learn about diabetes and a lot to learn about yourself. Changes like taking insulin and drinking fewer sweet drinks show that you have started a new lifestyle. Getting used to one change at a time can reduce your feelings of being overwhelmed about having diabetes.

4 How to find time to manage diabetes. Make a list of your new diabetes tasks. Don't forget to include relaxation as a new task. Share your list with family and ask how they can help in the home, so that you can have personal time to look after your needs — you can do this.

5 Be realistic. Plan one day at a time. Changes take time, months and even years.

6 Reach out to those who listen to you. Keep talking with health workers, family and friends. Let them help you with ideas to reduce your feelings of being overwhelmed. When you feel supported, you will feel better.

7 Remember to laugh. Diabetes is part of your life, but your life is still yours. Be with those who make you laugh because that always feels good. Watch your favorite comedy shows.

8 Walk away from stress. Your happy hormones (endorphins) flow through your body when you walk or exercise. A short 15-minute walk at any time of the day will give you energy to complete a task and feel better about yourself.

9 A positive attitude. Think about what you do well. Be proud of your work. Accept compliments. Say to yourself, "I can do this," to inspire you to make healthy changes for yourself.

10 **Commit to your better health.** All changes you make are entirely your choice and responsibility. Only you can change you. With supports and information, there is great hope for positive change and living well with diabetes.

Move More Sit Less

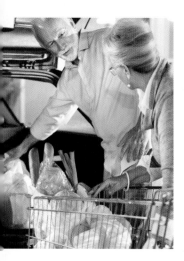

1 One step at a time. Park at the furthest spot at the grocery store and walk the extra distance. When you push a full grocery cart across the parking lot, that's a whole-body workout! Think about how important your health is, and how important *you* are. And enjoy the rewards of being active.

2 Fit walking into a busy schedule. When sitting at the computer or watching TV, stand up every hour and move around for a few minutes. If you replace half an hour of screen time every day with half an hour of exercise, you will be fitter and your blood sugar will improve.

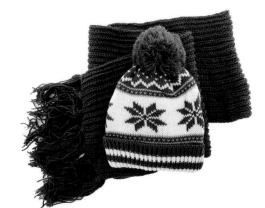

3 Keep active when it's cold or hot out. Dress in layers in the winter, and carry an umbrella on a hot day. Walk where the temperature is the same year round: a mall, hockey arena, your apartment hallways or your basement stairs.

4 Keep walking interesting. Listen to music or walk with a friend and you will walk further. Walk a new route for a change.

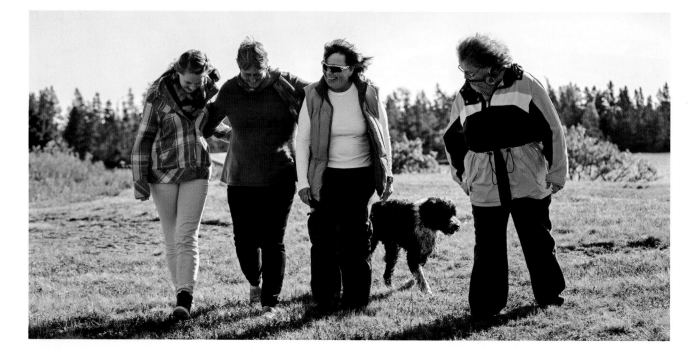

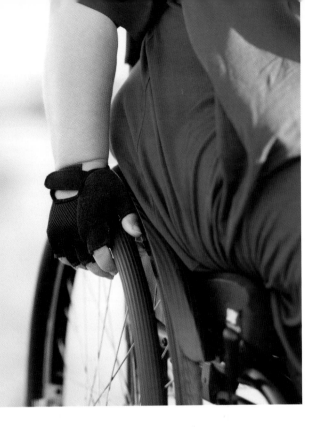

5 **Keep active in a wheelchair.** Gradually increase your wheeling pace and distance. Ask a physiotherapist to guide you in exercises. Find out about using a table top mini-exerciser for your arms. This improves your blood circulation.

6 **Take weight off your sore joints.** Use Nordic walking poles, a walker, walking cane or shopping cart and you will not get so tired. Or try swimming or water aerobics. If your legs become swollen after exercise, lie down and lift them up and rest them on pillows for 10 minutes. Take pain pills as prescribed.

7 **Warm up and cool down.** Walk comfortably for the first few minutes. Gently increase your walking pace. Slow down for the last few minutes of your walk.

8 **Avoid a low blood sugar episode.** Carry glucose tablets and take them if you feel light-headed.

9 **Protect your feet.** Wear socks and supportive, well-fitting shoes. Check your feet after your walk. Look for red spots and blisters. Stretch your toes apart and bend them up and down and do ankle circles to relieve foot cramps.

10 **When ready, move more.** Take longer walks, ride a bike or go to a gym and use a treadmill or elliptical machine. It's challenging but it gets easier. You have the power to improve your health.

When you bike, there is less weight on sore joints.

Sleep Well

1 **A good sleep improves diabetes.** Seven to 8 hours is recommended for adults; 8 to 10 hours for teenagers. Recommended sleep helps insulin work better night and day. But too little or too much sleep lowers your metabolism and disrupts your appetite hormones, which can result in weight gain. With a good sleep your body is recharged and ready to go.

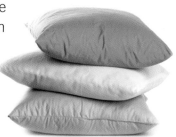

2 **Walk after supper.** It helps with digestion. Walking helps tire you out. Hormones (endorphins) are released while you walk to help you relax and get ready for sleep.

3 **Alcohol disrupts a sound sleep.** Also, drinking before bedtime can wake you up in the middle of the night to go pee.

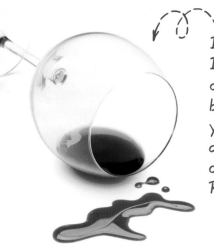

Did you know? Drinking alcohol before bed reduces your important dream phase of sleep (called REM sleep).

4 **Nicotine is a stimulant.** Nicotine increases your heart rate, blood pressure and brain activity. This can make it difficult to fall asleep and can disrupt sleep.

Try to have your last smoke an hour or two before bed. Better sleep is a good reason to think about quitting.

5 **No large bedtime snacks.** Most people do not need an evening snack to prevent low blood sugar at night. If you are having lows, talk to your doctor about adjusting your medications. If you are hungry, try snacks that are high in fiber and protein but not too high in carbohydrates. Limit large drinks of fluids.

6 **Fifteen minutes before your bedtime routine, turn off electronics.** This includes TV and checking social media. Your brain and eyes need time to shut down.

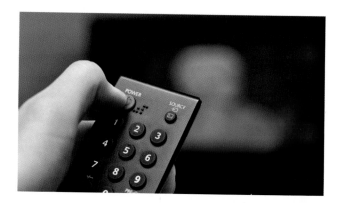

7 **Keep your bedroom cool, dark and quiet.** A good sleeping temperature is 18°C (65°F). Set your thermostat. Cover your windows with heavy, lined drapes or a blanket to reduce sounds and light.

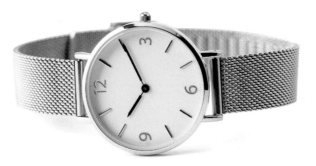

8 **Comfortable sleeping.** Is your mattress comfortable? Help your sore back with a pillow under your knees or between your knees. Wear warm loose socks if your feet get cold.

10 **Regular bedtime gives you a regular wake-up time.** This means you will have a regular breakfast time, which is an important start to managing diabetes every day.

9 **Just like children, we all need a bedtime routine.** Establish your own relaxing routine that works for you and stick with it. Brush your teeth and do a calming activity. Take a shower, moisturize your skin or read a book. Give thanks for a positive event of the day.

Manage Diabetes Nerve Pain

1 Understanding diabetes nerve damage (neuropathy). Healthy blood vessels bring nutrients and oxygen to your nerves. Years of high blood sugar damages blood vessels and nerve cells. Damaged nerves can cause either pain or loss of feeling.

2 What are symptoms of nerve pain? The pain is typically in feet, legs, hands or arms, especially at night. It may be sharp, burning, throbbing, or give you a cramp. A numb or tingly feeling can be as bothersome as pain. Rate your pain on a scale of 1 to 10 and let your doctor know.

3 You must reduce your blood sugar to reduce or stop diabetes nerve pain. Try to make even small changes and remember you may need a change to your diabetes medications.

4 Proven benefit of exercise. Exercise increases circulation so blood can carry more oxygen and nutrients to your nerves. Nerves can heal and this can reduce pain in the long term.

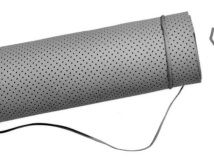

(((Trying yoga for the first time? Go slow and easy — don't be pressured to overstretch.

5 To help manage pain when exercising. Do low impact exercise. For walking, you might find it helpful to wear socks that are padded on the bottom, or put gel inserts in your shoes. Be sure your shoes still have enough room to wiggle your toes. Poor balance may be related to nerve damage in your feet. Swimming or water aerobics might be helpful.

6 Use a bed cradle at night. This attaches to the bottom of your bed so you can lift the sheets and blankets off your legs and feet. A pair of loose socks will keep your feet warm.

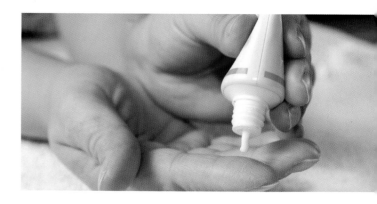

7 Medicated creams, patches and pills. Capsaicin cream and lidocaine skin patches help some people with their neuropathy pain. Ibuprofen (Aspirin and Advil) reduce inflammation. Acetaminophen (Tylenol) reduces chemical pain signals to the brain. Alpha-lipoic acid and CBD topical creams (hemp products) are new to the market. Always check with your doctor about the safety of over-the-counter medications for you.

8 **A physiotherapist or pain clinic.** Here, you may receive TENS therapy: small pads are placed on your skin at the site of the pain, and a machine sends small electrical impulses. Other options include stretching exercises, biofeedback (a relaxation technique), hypnosis, acupressure and acupuncture.

10 **Prescription pain pills.** Codeine is prescription only. Your doctor may prescribe it for urgent short-term use. Pills typically given for depression or convulsions (epilepsy) may also work to suppress pain in nerves. Your doctor may suggest medical cannabis as an option that may have fewer side effects than some other drugs.

9 **Manage nerve pain with relaxation or distraction.** Watch a meditative video, or close your eyes, relax and listen to meditative music. Hormones are released when you relax, which helps reduce pain. Try gentle massage or a warm or cold wrap for short periods of time.

Protect Your Eyes

1 **Retinopathy — no early warning signs.** This is when years of high blood sugar and high blood pressure damage the tiny blood vessels in your retina (the back of your eye). It is a major cause of diabetes-related blindness, but treatment — especially early treatment — can delay or prevent this.

2 **Get a dilated eye exam every year.** This is to check for retinopathy as well as macular degeneration and glaucoma.

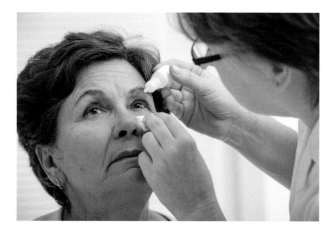

3 **If your vision becomes blurry.** This does not necessarily mean retinopathy. This may be due to changes in your blood sugar level that causes the lens of your eyes to swell and shrink. Your optometrist will not prescribe new glasses until your blood sugar stabilizes.

4 **Sudden changes in your vision.** See an eye doctor right away if you have sudden loss of vision in one or both eyes, flashing lights, spots or floaters of any color, or double vision.

5 **How to prevent or reduce eye damage.** As a person with diabetes you must reduce your high blood sugar, high blood pressure and blood cholesterol. You must also consider cutting back smoking and consider drinking less alcohol.

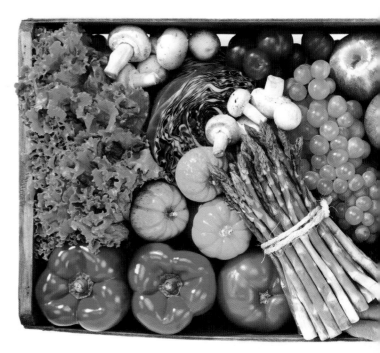

6 **Food for your eyes.** Dark green, orange and yellow vegetables and fruits have excellent vitamins and minerals to maintain healthy eyes. Eat fish for omega-3 fats and eggs for lutein.

7 **Dry eyes and diabetes.** Diabetes nerve damage to tear ducts makes your eyes dry. Take extra caution if you wear contact lenses, as you are more at risk of dry eye as well as eye infections.

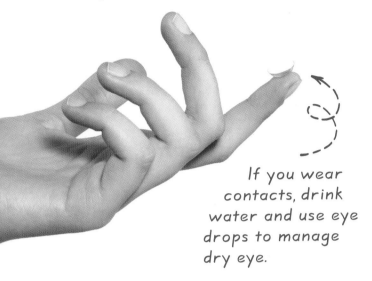

If you wear contacts, drink water and use eye drops to manage dry eye.

8 **Wear sunglasses outdoors all year round.** As a person with diabetes you are more likely to get cataracts. UV sunglasses help slow the development of cataracts and other eye diseases.

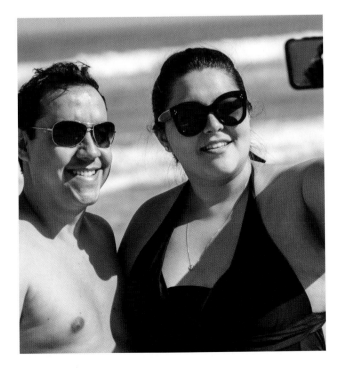

9 **Wear protective safety glasses to avoid eye injuries.** A small object could fly into your eye when you cut the grass, or drill, grind, sand or saw. As a person with diabetes, if your eye is injured, it heals much slower and is more likely to get infected.

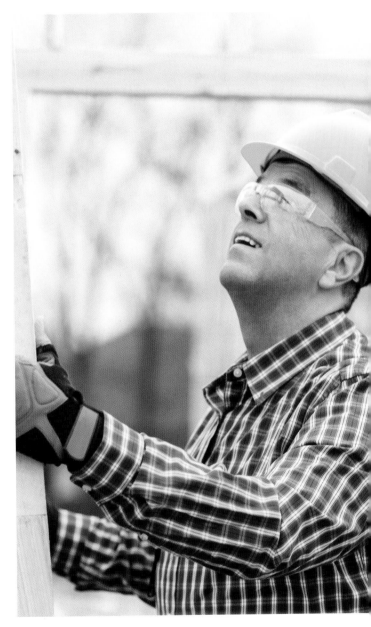

10 **Laser treatment may be required for more advanced retinopathy.** Lasers are tiny light beams directed into your eye to prevent more damage from retinopathy.

Care for Your Gums and Teeth

1 **What is gum disease?** Bacteria builds up on your gums and teeth as plaque, which can cause tender, bleeding gums and infection. Gum disease is the leading cause of tooth loss in adults.

2 **Diabetes and gum disease.** High blood sugar may cause an infection of your gums. Once gums are infected, blood sugar can go even higher.

3 **Act now to reduce high blood sugar.** If you have gum disease, your doctor needs to know. You will need to start on insulin or increase insulin or try a new medication to bring down your blood sugar. Mouth infections take a longer time to heal with diabetes.

4 **Healthy food for your teeth and gums.** Choose milk, cheese, yogurt, fruits and vegetables. Fiber helps to stimulate your gums and keep them firm. Extra chewing increases saliva that neutralizes mouth bacteria. Eat fewer sugary and sweet foods and drinks.

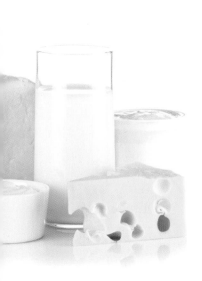

5 **Exercise helps your teeth and gums.** Exercise improves blood flow, immunity and blood sugar. Blood vessels and nerves in your mouth will be healthier.

6 **Smoking and gum disease.** Nicotine from cigarettes or vaping narrows blood vessels and can reduce your body's ability to fight infections. Nicotine also decreases insulin action.

7 **Drink water throughout the day.** People with diabetes often make less saliva and have dry mouth. Sipping water during the day helps. After you eat or drink soft drinks or other beverages, rinse with water to wash away acids and sugars.

8 **See your dental hygienist once or twice a year.** This is the time for cleaning, checking for cavities and to see if you have early signs of gum disease. Tell the hygienist about any pain in your mouth. Go sooner if you think you have an infection.

9 **Brush and floss your teeth.** Gently brush twice a day and floss before bedtime. Rough brushing or flossing can damage your gums. Use a soft or extra soft toothbrush or an electric toothbrush. Rinse your mouth well with water after you brush and floss.

10 **Care for your dentures.** Take them out every night; this gives your gums a chance to rest. Brush and rinse your dentures as often as you can through the day. The denturist will explain how to properly care for them.

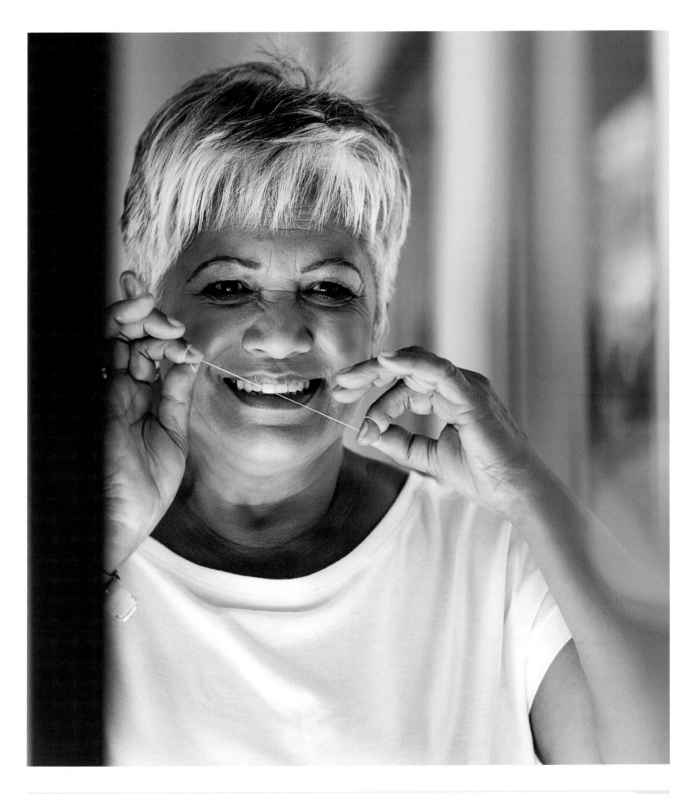

Your Heart and Blood Vessels

1 **Narrow blood vessels.** High blood sugar over time causes extra fat in the blood. This thickens and narrows all blood vessels, which reduces blood flow and increases blood pressure. Your heart and brain can be harmed, as well as your kidneys, eyes and feet.

2 **Higher risk for heart attack and stroke.** When a blood vessel to the heart is blocked it can cause a heart attack. When a blood vessel in the brain is blocked it can cause a stroke. Early treatment means better outcomes.

3 **ACR blood test measures risk for heart attack and stroke.** This test shows if your kidneys are leaking protein into your urine, which means your blood vessels may be narrowing. Other early signs might be unusual shortness of breath, calf pain, chest pain or headaches.

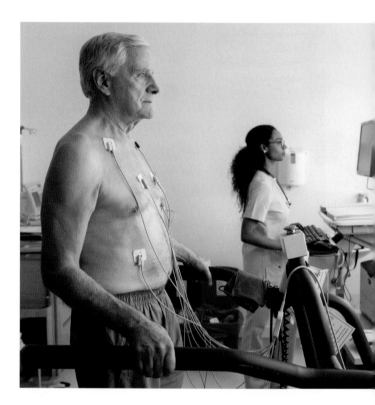

4 **A follow-up ECG test.** This may be ordered if your ACR is elevated. It shows your heart rate and whether you have a heart problem.

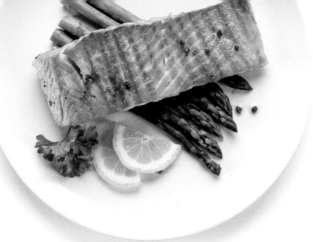

5 **What you can do to help your heart.** Eat healthier food. Cut down on portions of food to lose weight. Walk and exercise regularly. Exercise slowly with care to protect your heart. Manage your stress. Quit smoking. Take your medications regularly.

6 **How your doctor can help you.** By prescribing medications; possibly two or more heart pills. Let your doctor know if you have any side effects. Your doctor will also monitor your lab results.

7 **Warning signs of a heart attack.** Immediately seek help if you have:

- sudden tightness or pain in your chest, neck, jaw, shoulder, arms or back, that lasts more than a few minutes
- chest pain when you exert yourself
- shortness of breath
- nausea, indigestion or vomiting
- sudden sweating
- unusual fear or anxiety

Don't take symptoms lightly. Every second counts. If you are having a heart attack, early treatment can reduce damage to your heart muscle. Immediately dial 911 and chew a 325 mg aspirin.

8 **Warning signs of a stroke.** If you have these symptoms, immediately seek help:

V – Vision loss, sudden
F – Face drooping
A – Arm weakness
S – Speech slurred
T – Time to call 911

9 **Open-heart bypass surgery.** It is like a road detour where doctors close off the blocked vessel and bypass into another blood vessel around the blocked vessel.

10 **Angioplasty heart surgery.** This involves a tube inserted through a groin artery as far as the blockage. A balloon at the end of the tube is enlarged, causing the artery to widen. Usually a stent (a metal tube) is then placed in the artery to keep it open.

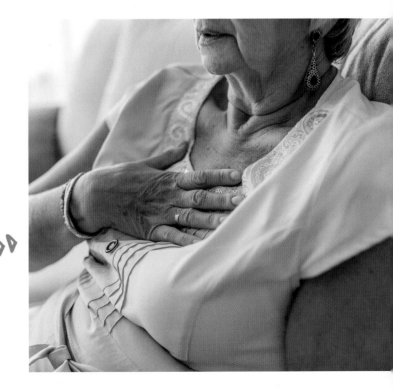

Let's Talk About Smoking

1 **Nicotine is a toxic substance.** Nicotine is responsible for increasing the risk of every single diabetes complication. Now is the time to think about quitting.

Did you know? Over 50 chemicals that can cause cancer come from a burning cigarette.

2 **E-cigarettes are not a quit-smoking aid.** They have nicotine just like cigarettes and in some cases have more. Using them may be called vaping or juuling.

3 **Educate yourself.** Talk to your doctor, pharmacist or diabetes educator. Read the quit-smoking pamphlets. Call a toll-free quit line counselor — they will be there 24/7 by phone to help and support you.

4 **Nicotine replacement therapy (NRT).** It has been proven that when you use NRT you are more likely to quit smoking for good. NRT gives you controlled doses of nicotine, which are lessened over time. Examples are the nicotine patch, inhaler and sprays, gums and lozenges.

5 **Medications and other treatments.** There are quit-smoking prescription pills for heavy smokers. Find out about hypnosis, acupuncture or laser therapy.

6 **Set a quit date.** You may want to reduce slowly to your quit date. Every cigarette you don't smoke is a fantastic step forward in the right direction. Remember to use nicotine gum or lozenges as you start to cut back.

7 **Control cravings.** Nicotine withdrawal is a whole body and mind reaction. **D**elay, Breathe **D**eeply, **D**rink Water and **D**istract Yourself. This will help you get through each craving one at a time. You will find strengths about yourself you didn't know.

8 **Irritability.** When you feel frustrated and anxious with people or situations, try to get away and take the time to calm down.

9 **Prevent weight gain.** If you were a pack-a-day smoker — you puffed on a cigarette up to 300 times a day (12 puffs per smoke). You don't want to exchange that with food and drink. Stock your kitchen with low-calorie food and healthy snacks. Practice mindful eating and foods will start to taste more flavorful and interesting.

10 **Easy to say — hard to do.**
It may take several tries
before you quit for good. There
are good resources to support
you. Keep them close at hand.
After you quit smoking you will
discover you want to eat better
and walk more and really enjoy
the wonders of feeling healthy.

Probiotics and Prebiotics

Probiotics

1 **What are probiotics?** Probiotics are gut bacteria. There are hundreds of different kinds of probiotic bacteria that live in your large intestine and digest food. These "good bacteria" work together to keep you healthy. They are found in yogurt and other fermented foods.

2 **Why are probiotics important for diabetes?** While digesting food, probiotic bacteria slow down blood sugar rise after a meal. They also help build a strong immune system. They send chemical messages to your brain to help control appetite. These bacteria even help determine how many calories or nutrients you get from food.

3 **Did you know? Antibiotics kill these good bacteria.** Antibiotics reduce infections, but they also kill some of the probiotic bacteria in your gut. So, if you're taking antibiotics, eat foods that are rich in probiotic bacteria. And keep eating them after you finish the antibiotics, to restore your gut health.

4 **Breastfeeding and probiotics.** New research shows that human milk has probiotics. When a baby breastfeeds, special probiotic bacteria from the mother's milk get established in the baby's gut and stay there for life. Breastfed babies get fewer infections and therefore need less antibiotics.

PROBIOTIC FOODS

5 **Fermented milks.** Yogurt, buttermilk and sour cream are types of fermented milk. Some cheeses such as Gouda, Cheddar, Swiss, Parmesan and cottage cheese are also in this group. So are popular fermented drinks such as kefir from Russia and the Middle East, and ayran from Turkey.

6 **Other fermented foods.** These include sauerkraut, sourdough bread, pickles and olives, soy sauce and Worcestershire sauce. Kimchi (made from cabbage and radishes) and miso and tempeh (made from soybeans) are popular Asian fermented foods. Most of these foods have strong or sour flavors. Caution: most of them are high in salt.

Sauerkraut

Some types of cheese, such as Parmesan and Gouda

Olives

Buttermilk

Prebiotics

7 **What are prebiotics?** They are soluble-fiber foods. They play a significant role because soluble fiber is the food that probiotic bacteria eat. It allows the "good bacteria" to grow and multiply in your gut.

PREBIOTIC FOODS

8 **Raw vegetables and whole fruits.** Fruits and vegetables are always healthy. When you eat them raw, they have more unbroken fiber and more enzymes, which healthy probiotic bacteria grow on.

9 **Foods with inulin, a special type of soluble fiber.** Inulin fiber is found in jicama, onions, leeks, garlic, asparagus, barley and dark rye bread. If you were thinking to cut back on coffee, a natural substitute is roasted chicory root beverage. Chicory root is especially high in inulin.

10 **Beans and lentils.** Include them at least once a week in your meals and you will increase fiber in your gut for probiotic bacteria to thrive on. Try Lentil Spinach Soup (page 71), Split Pea Soup (page 76), Vegetarian Chili (page 92) and Taco Bean Salad Dinner (page 97).

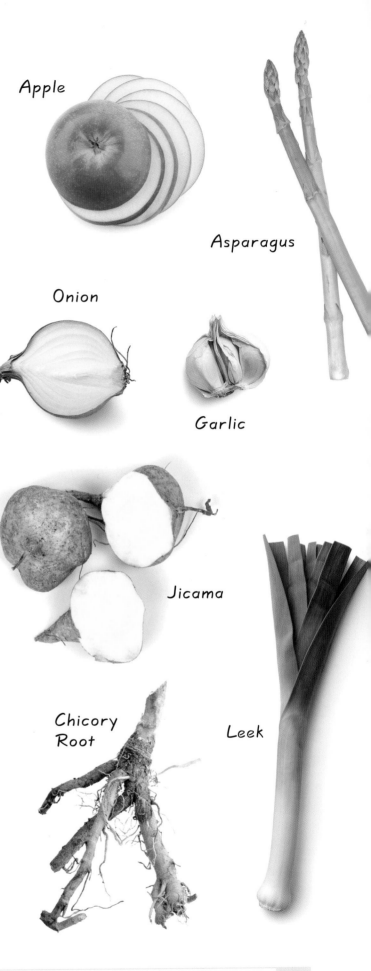

Apple

Asparagus

Onion

Garlic

Jicama

Chicory Root

Leek

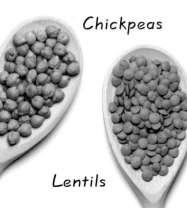

Chickpeas

Lentils

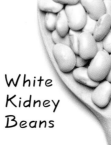

White Kidney Beans

Relieve Constipation

1 **Why does diabetes cause constipation, or make it worse?** High blood sugar over many years damages the nerves that contract your bowel muscles. Constipation can also be caused by lack of fiber in your diet, too little exercise, too much stress, and side-effects from medications.

2 **What does "regular" mean?** Good regularity means you go daily, or every second or third day. Your stool should be soft and easy to pass.

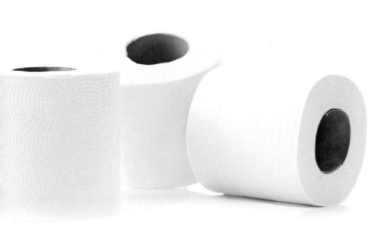

3 **Regular time to sit on the toilet.** Allow time in the morning to eat your breakfast, which may provide an urge for a bowel movement before you leave home.

4 **Slowly add more fiber to your meals.** Try rye or whole wheat bread and whole grain crackers. Choose brown rice, whole wheat pasta, oatmeal, All-Bran and Shredded Wheat, bran muffins, beans and lentils, barley, and nuts and seeds. Sprinkle flax seeds, chia seeds or 100% bran on your cereals, yogurt, soups, casseroles, mashed potatoes and salads.

Try the recipe for Slim Bits made with chia seeds on page 111.

5 **Eat five or more vegetables and fruits each day.** Try vegetables at breakfast: tomatoes, sliced cucumbers or spinach with your eggs. Include at least two vegetables at lunch and dinner. Have a fruit for an afternoon snack.

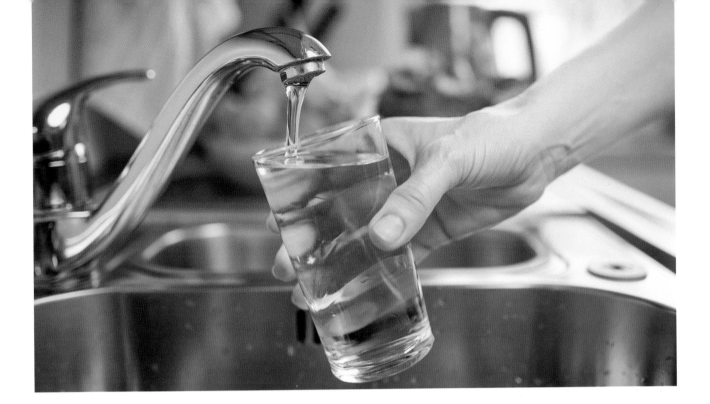

6 **Drink water throughout the day.** As you eat more fiber, you must drink more water to keep your stool soft. Try to drink six or more cups of water a day. A cup of hot water first thing in the morning can help.

7 **The value of a daily walk.** Walking strengthens bowel muscles and reduces constipation. The bowel contracts and then relaxes as you walk, and this helps form a stool.

8 **Exercises that help relieve constipation.** For each exercise, lie on your back with your knees bent. Do each exercise five times.

- **PELVIC TILT:** Tighten your stomach muscles and push your back into the bed. Breathe, and hold for five seconds.
- **LEG PULL-UP:** Place your hands under your knee and bring your leg towards your chest. Hold for five seconds, then return your leg to the bent position. Repeat with your other leg.

9 **Prunes.** Prunes have fiber and a type of sugar called sorbitol, which is a laxative. Try not to depend on prunes every day as your laxative. Eat different high fiber fruits on different days and this will also help increase your healthy gut bacteria.

2 prunes or ¹/₄ cup prune juice is equal to 1 fruit 〉〉〉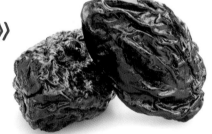

10 **Stool softeners or laxatives.** Talk to your doctor about the safe use of one of these: mineral oil, sugar-free Metamucil, Milk of Magnesia, Ex-lax, Dulcolax or MiraLAX, suppository or enema. A cup of herbal senna tea is a milder laxative. These are for short-term use only, to avoid dependency.

Kidneys and Diabetes

1 **Diabetes is the main cause of chronic kidney disease.** Chronic kidney disease is the gradual loss of kidney function caused by high blood sugar and high blood pressure.

2 **ACR is an important urine test.** This measures small amounts of protein that have leaked into the urine. It is an early sign of kidney damage. When you are first diagnosed with diabetes you will have this urine test, and then once every year.

3 **eGFR is an important blood test.** This measures the rate at which your kidneys filter blood. A lower eGFR means low kidney function. The doctor will not determine kidney function based on one blood test. Several blood tests will likely be ordered.

4 **Keep active.** Exercise improves blood circulation through the kidney's tiny filters. Kidneys have millions of tiny tubes that filter waste out of the blood.

5 **Alcohol.** Alcohol in the body raises blood pressure. High blood pressure damages the filters in your kidneys. Think about your kidneys every time you have a drink!

6 **Smoking.** Nicotine hardens and narrows blood vessels, which increases blood pressure. As with alcohol, nicotine is a toxic chemical that damages the kidneys.

7 **Salt.** When kidneys are damaged they no longer filter out all the salt from the foods you eat. This means the salt builds up in your blood. This can increase your blood pressure and worsen swelling in your legs and feet. Cut back on salt and continue to drink clean water to flush out your kidneys.

8 **Potassium and phosphorus.** When kidneys are damaged they no longer filter out all the potassium and phosphorus. These nutrients are naturally present in many foods and are often added to processed foods. If your lab results show that you have excess amounts of potassium and phosphorus, your dietitian will suggest diet changes.

9 **Kidneys work hard to filter medications.** So make sure you just take the ones you need. Ask your doctor to do a review. There may be some pills — such as Advil, vitamins or herbal supplements — that you should stop taking.

10 **Sick day medication list.** Tell your doctor if you are ill with vomiting or diarrhea. Some of your diabetes medications or other medications may be stopped, to protect your kidneys until you feel better.

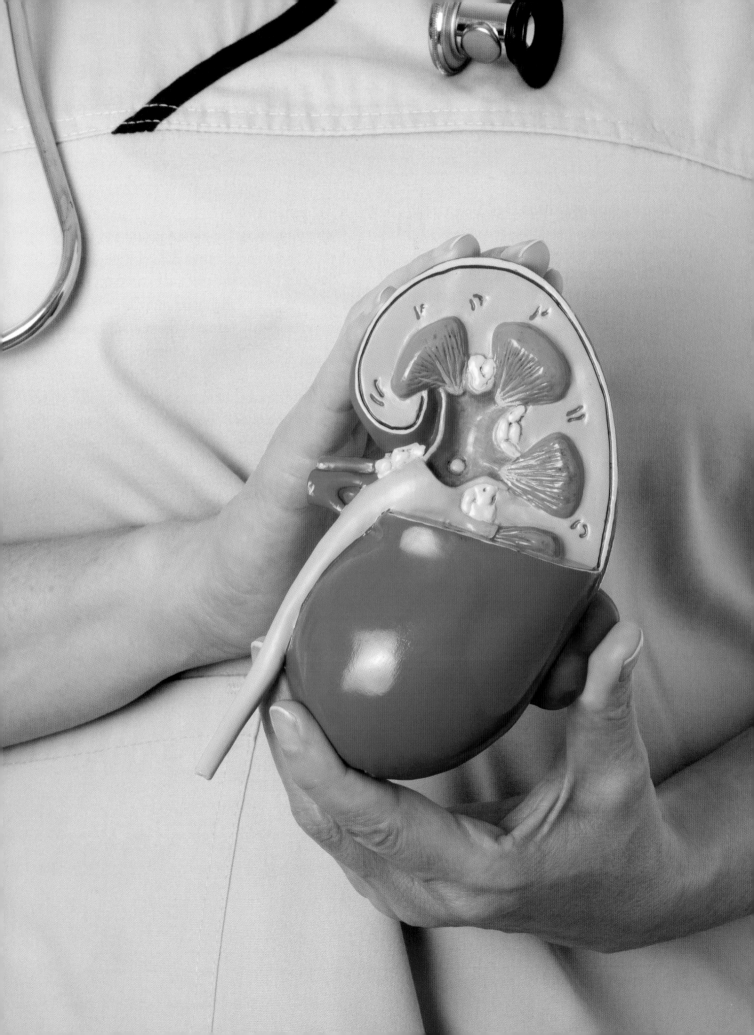

Manage Urinary Tract Infections

1 **What is a urinary tract infection (UTI)?** Also known as a bladder infection or kidney infection. This is when unhealthy bacteria or yeast grow in the urinary tract.

2 **Blood sugar has to come down.** As a person with diabetes, high blood sugar is your most common reason for a UTI. Once your bladder and kidneys are infected this can cause blood sugar to go even higher.

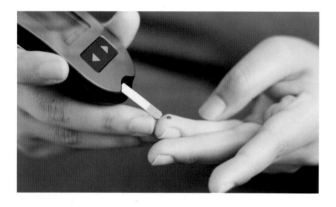

3 **Other causes of a UTI.** Consider these causes:

- If the bladder is not completely emptied, bacteria remain and grow into an infection.
- The diabetes medications known as SGLT2 inhibitors transport extra blood sugar into the urine and can also contribute to UTI.
- Kidney stones, catheter-use and poor hygiene are known causes of UTI.
- Women tend to have more UTI's than men. After peeing, women should wipe front to back so germs are not spread.

4 **Symptoms of a UTI.** You will feel the need to pee more often or urgently and it may sting. You may notice your urine smells or looks different. You could have stomach cramps or back pain.

5 **Drink water and pee regularly.** Water keeps your kidneys and bladder flushed out and clean. With diabetes nerve damage, and for men with an enlarged prostate, you may not feel whether your bladder has been completely emptied. Pee every two hours during the day and empty your bladder fully.

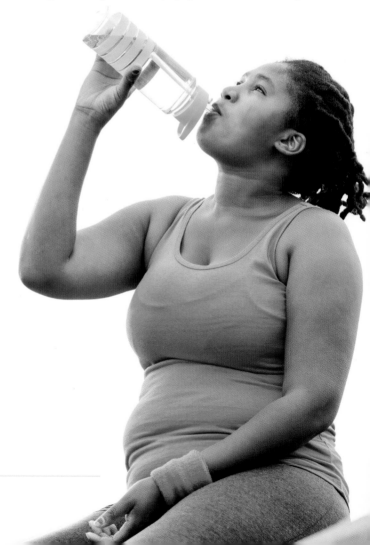

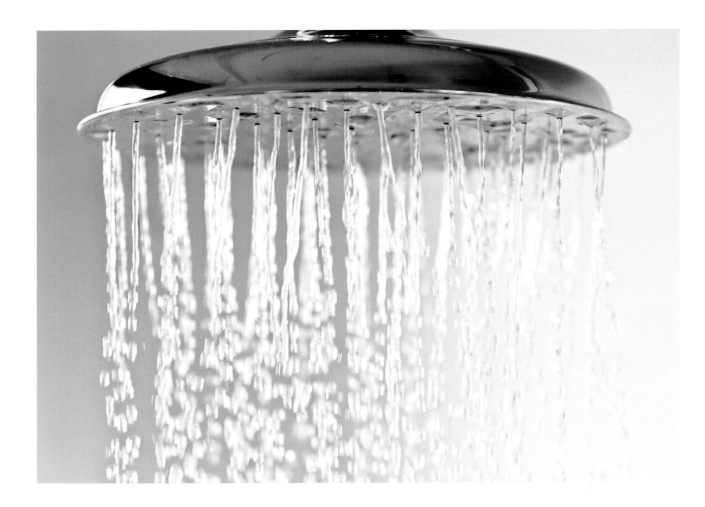

6 **Clean body.** A warm shower is a better choice than soaking in a bathtub. Avoid perfumed soaps, and dry well after your shower. Change menstrual pads or inserts and incontinence pads regularly.

7 **Clean sex.** To help prevent a UTI, wash before and after sex so you are both clean. And always pee after sex to clear germs out of the urethra.

8 **Get a urine test.** Depending on how serious the infection is, women may need a pelvic exam (similar to a pap test) and men may be given a rectal exam to check the size of the prostate gland.

9 **What medication is prescribed?** The doctor will order medication based on your symptoms. Antibiotics are prescribed for bacterial infections. If your doctor knows your health issues well, you may get a prescription over the phone. If you feel better before you have finished the antibiotic prescription, you must still complete the treatment. Go back to your doctor if you do not get better.

10 **Yeast infections.** Antibiotics kill good bacteria with the bad. So, after being treated for a UTI, a woman may get a vaginal yeast infection or a man may get a penis yeast infection. Different medications will then be needed.

Refresh Your Sex Life

1 **Boost circulation and nerves between your legs.** Exercise also boosts nitric oxide in the blood system, which is known to help arouse our sex organs. Cut back on smoking because nicotine narrows your blood vessels, which reduces blood circulation and can reduce a man's erection.

2 **Check your medications.** Diuretics and blood pressure pills, antidepressants, sleeping pills, antihistamines, appetite suppressants, and drugs for ulcers or cancer may have side effects that cause low sexual desire or erectile dysfunction. Ask your doctor if there are other medications for you without this side effect.

3 **PDE5's (Viagra-type drugs) for men.** Sildenafil is the generic name for Viagra. Other PDE5's are vardenafil (Levitra), tadalafil (Cialis) and avanafil (Stendra). These often work for men with diabetes who are not able to get or maintain a firm erection. Start with the lowest dose (25 mg). For the pill to work properly it is important to take it about one hour before sex and on an empty stomach. Let your doctor know how it works for you, or if you have side effects such as headaches. If one type of PDE5 doesn't work, your doctor can suggest a different one or a different dose. You should not use PDE5's if you are on heart medicines known as nitrates.

4 **Other medications.** These include estrogen for women and testosterone for men, to help with various aspects of sexual health. Also, there are other erectile dysfunction medications if PDE5's aren't working. Always ask your doctor about drug benefits and side effects.

5 **Build intimacy.** Be kind, share in home duties and do fun things together. Go for a walk and hold hands. This all helps to build closeness and desire in the bedroom.

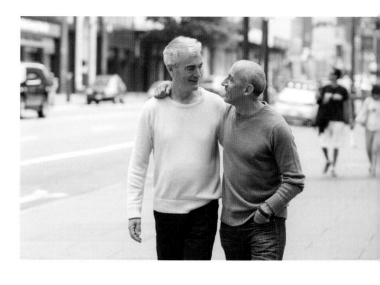

6 **Seduce each other.** If you'd like tonight to be the night, then schedule it. Send a text with a romantic tone to see if the interest is mutual. At home, prepare for your special night together, and turn down the lights.

The *Complete Diabetes Guide* (see page 192) has an extensive section on sexuality and diabetes.

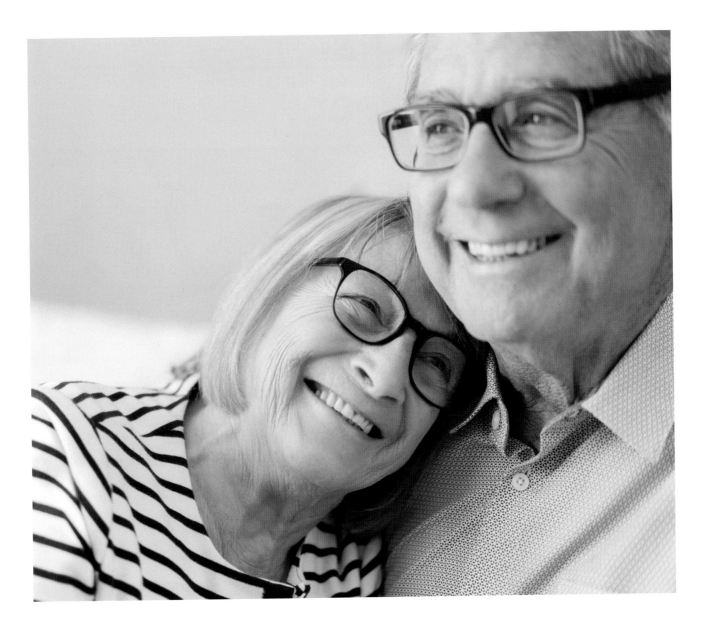

7 **Foreplay or after-play.** Make time for sensual foreplay, kissing, touching, caressing. Use water-based lubricants. If it's a quickie that works — enjoy intimate time after as well.

8 **Penis tension bands.** These are an easy and low-cost solution for men to maintain an erection. Place the right-sized band at the base of the penis once you start getting hard. Remove it if it hurts, and keep it on no longer than 30 minutes. For discretion, these can be ordered at major online stores.

9 **Try a new position.** Sore backs, sore hips and sore knees, means changing positions so you both feel comfortable. Use lots of pillows for support.

10 **Sexually transmitted infections.** STI's are spread through oral or genital contact with an infected partner. STI's include infections such as HIV and HPV virus, syphilis, and herpes from cold sores. Search online "STI hotline" for STI prevention information.

Help for Swollen Legs, Ankles and Feet

1 Move more. If you sit or stand for long periods of time in a day, fluids can settle in your legs, ankles and feet. To reduce this, take time to stretch, bend and walk around.

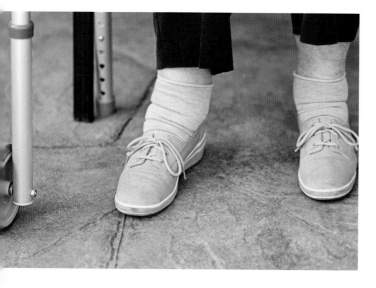

2 Stay out of the heat. When it is hot your blood vessels expand and more fluids settle in your legs, ankles and feet. People with diabetes may sweat less, due to nerve damage to their sweat glands. So their natural way to cool down is lost. A cold drink of water on a hot day is refreshing.

3 Raise your legs. Put your feet on a stool when you sit. Apply a cold cloth to reduce swelling. When you lie down, place a pillow under your feet so they are raised.

4 Your doctor may recommend compression socks or stockings. Start with a lightweight pair that are not too tight and are easier to put on and take off. These provide pain relief and help prevent fluids from collecting in your legs, ankles and feet.

5 Wear good shoes to protect your feet. When your feet and ankles swell, your shoes or socks can cut into your skin; a sore could then get infected. Shop for shoes at the end of the day when your feet are most swollen, to be sure of a wide enough fit.

6 Eat less salt. The body holds on to too much water when you eat too much salt. Cutting back on salt reduces swelling and many other health problems.

Use spices instead of salt to flavor your food.

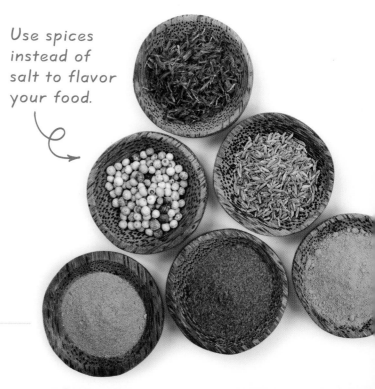

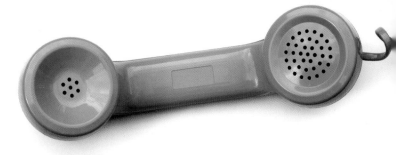

7 **Drink less alcohol.** Your body holds more water after drinking alcohol, which can worsen swollen legs, ankles and feet.

8 **Lose five pounds.** This takes weight off your legs and feet and will reduce swelling. You may feel so much better that you will be motivated to lose another five pounds.

9 **Medication review.** Prednisone, pioglitazone (a diabetes pill), some antidepressants, pain pills and blood pressure pills cause swelling as a side effect. Your doctor may prescribe diuretic medications to remove excess fluid, or a blood thinner if you are at risk of a blood clot.

10 **When to call your doctor.** Call your doctor if you have:

- Swelling that is new, sudden or gets worse
- Abnormal heartbeat, shortness of breath, chest pain
- An ulcer, broken skin, blister or infection on your foot or leg
- Swelling or redness on one side of your calf or leg. This could be a sign of a blood clot. If you have any trouble breathing, chest pain, pressure or tightness, it could mean the clot has moved up to your lungs or heart — call 911 immediately

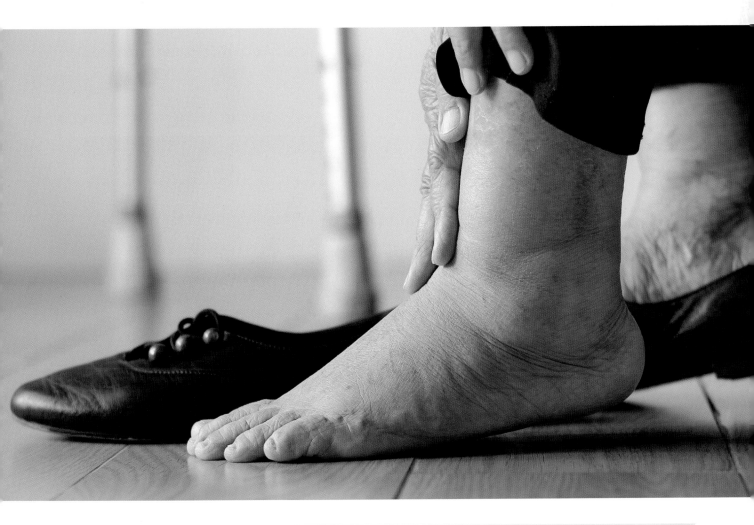

Healthy Feet for Life

1 **Losing feeling in your feet.** Diabetes nerve damage means you may not feel a cut on your foot. This cut can quickly become infected. Nerve damage also causes dry, cracked skin and it can even change the shape of your foot.

2 **Be responsible for your own feet.** Using a mirror can help you see the bottom of your feet. Look for redness, swelling, cracks, bleeding, corns and calluses and changes to your toenails. Wash small cuts and sores with soap and water. Cover them with a sterile bandage and check to make sure they are healing. With proper foot care and good blood sugar you can have healthy feet for life.

4 **Trim your toenails carefully.** Trim straight across; not too short. File any sharp edges. A qualified foot nurse can do the work if you cannot reach your feet.

Flat-edged nail clippers are recommended. →

5 **Do not use heaters, razors or chemicals.** If your feet get cold, do not use electric blankets or hot water bottles filled with boiling water. Instead, put on wooly socks. Do not scrape off dead skin with razors or knives and do not use corn plasters or other chemicals on your feet.

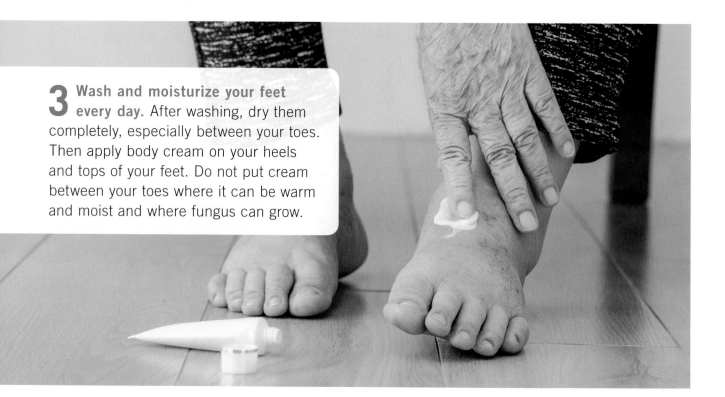

3 **Wash and moisturize your feet every day.** After washing, dry them completely, especially between your toes. Then apply body cream on your heels and tops of your feet. Do not put cream between your toes where it can be warm and moist and where fungus can grow.

6 **Wear comfortable socks.** Cotton and wool socks are best. Try merino wool, which is naturally anti-bacterial, breathable and warm. They may cost more but your feet are worth it. Choose light colored ones so you will see if there is a sore that is bleeding.

7 **Buy shoes that fit well.** As a person with diabetes, a proper fitting pair of shoes is one of the most important investments you will make. You may have to shop at a specialty shoe store. Ask the salesperson for shoes with a deep toe box so your toes will not rub together.

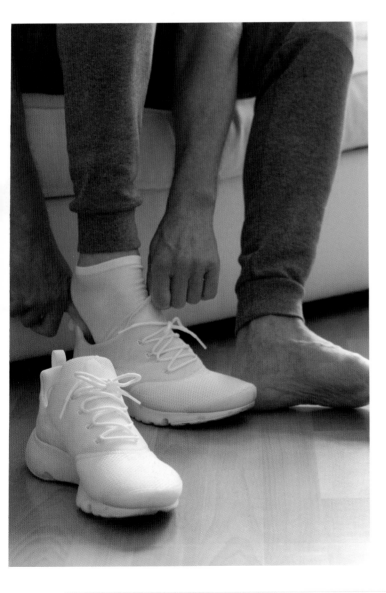

No butts about it! Smoking is bad for your feet.

8 **Stop smoking.** The nicotine in cigarettes is extremely damaging to your blood vessels. It narrows blood vessels, which prevents normal blood flow to your feet. Less blood flow means less oxygen and nutrients to the nerve cells. When the nerve cells are not working well, you lose feeling in your feet or experience pain in your feet.

9 **Ask your doctor or nurse to check your feet.** They can check the pulse in your feet and the sensation on the bottom of your feet. Don't be shy — at least once a year, have your feet checked in their office.

10 **Urgent foot problems?** See your doctor if a foot or toenail sore doesn't heal within two days. Or, if swelling or redness in your feet or legs does not go away in two days. See your doctor sooner if it quickly worsens or you are concerned.

Amputations aren't as common as they used to be — but they're still real, they still happen. That's why foot care is crucial. Follow all 10 of these steps, and almost all diabetes-related foot and leg amputations can be prevented.

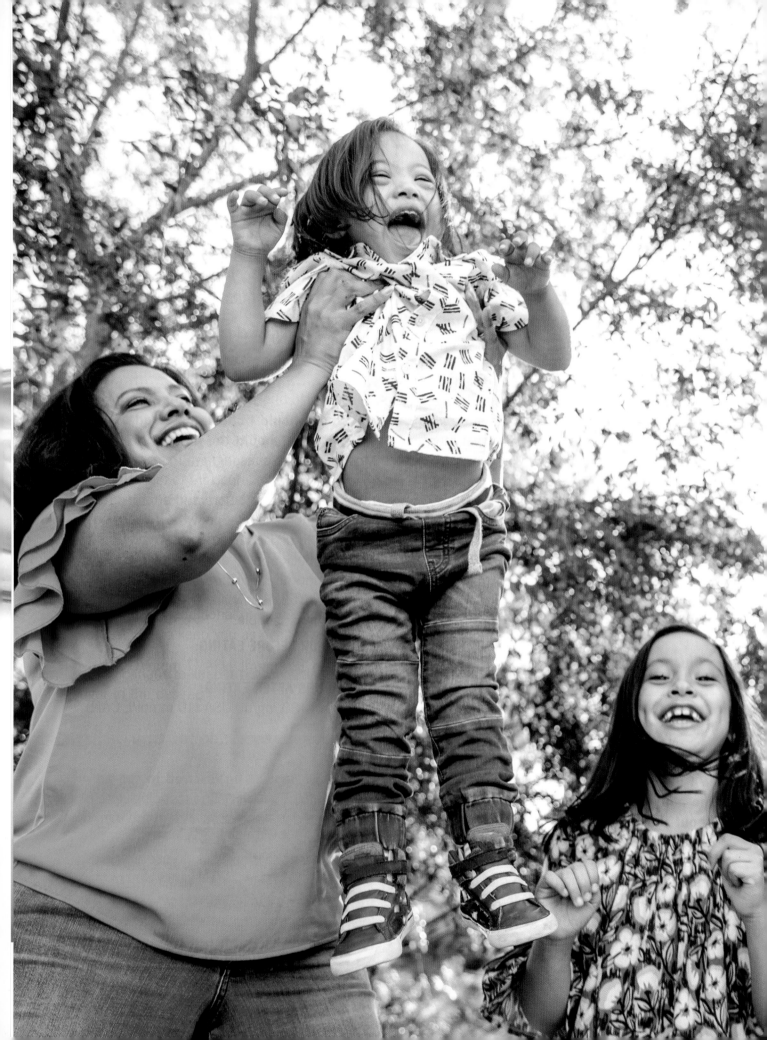

Diabetes Health for All Ages

Diabetes and Families

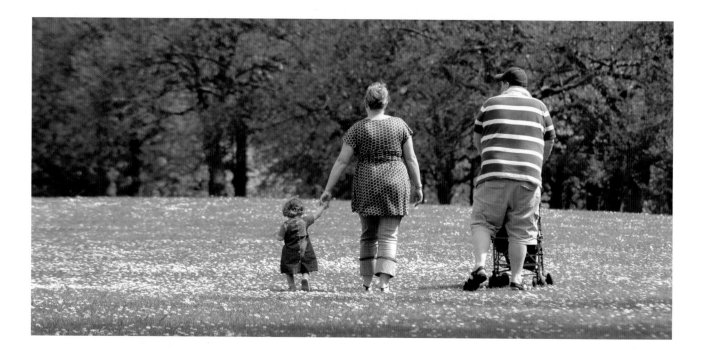

1 Health of your family. You are choosing a healthy lifestyle to manage your diabetes, which will make a positive difference for your whole family. A healthy lifestyle can delay and sometimes prevent diabetes for your family members.

2 Time to work together to find a common goal. As you make changes, you may find that no one in your family wants to change along with you. Involve them in what you are learning. Become their teacher in diabetes management. They need to know you are serious about your changes and they will learn to respect you for your commitment to improve every family member's health.

3 Family support. Ask your family how they feel about your diagnosis and how it has affected them. Everyone needs to be heard. Then you can talk about supporting each other.

4 Other family changes. Your diagnosis will affect your family. Just like other changes you may be going through — loss of work, moves, marriage, deaths, divorce or retirement. Be prepared for the time it is going to take to manage the changes of a new lifestyle living with diabetes.

Like a butterfly, take time to rest and take flight when you are ready.

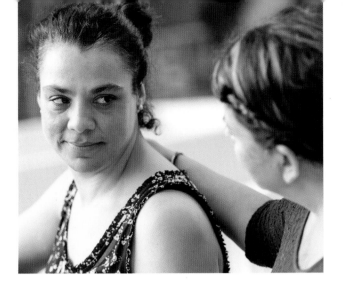

7 Five Stages of Change for you and your family. Change is not a simple process. Change involves effort, which takes time. Many people go back and forth through the five stages before they make a lasting change in behavior. The five stages of change are not being ready, getting ready, being ready for change, actually making a change and then maintaining the change.

5 Shifts in mood. Large shifts in your blood sugar levels can make you irritated or angry. Mood swings are usually short-lived. Let your family know this.

8 Build your self-confidence. It can be overwhelming trying to sort out your new life and family situation now that you have been diagnosed with a chronic disease. If you feel sadness or emotional pain, this may be a good time to try professional counseling. It helps some people move past blame and self-blame, and helps them set positive goals.

6 Five Stages of Grief for you and your family. When you are diagnosed with diabetes, you have to give up many things that you love such as favorite foods in large portions. This is a loss in your life and you will grieve and so will your family. This is how many people respond to grief or loss: denial, anger, bargaining, depression and acceptance. The five stages of grief are normal and help explain the emotions you and your family are feeling.

9 Diabetes can mean positive change for your family. If you used to eat on-the-go, more home cooking and sharing of meals can lead to more talk and laughter. When you go for walks together this becomes a special time to talk about the day. Over time, family will adjust and the changes will become the new normal.

10 Families have the greatest influence on children. A caring, supportive home helps a child grow up healthy (less likely to smoke, drink or take drugs). It also helps the child be emotionally strong (self-confident and mature) and physically fit and energetic. This means less diabetes.

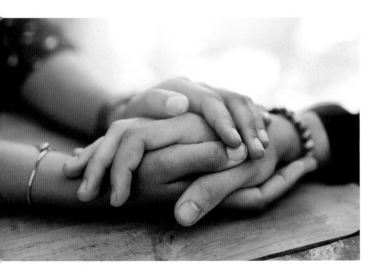

Diabetes and Families **153**

Budgeting for Diabetes

1 **The cost of managing diabetes.** There are many new expenses for a person who has been diagnosed with type 2 diabetes. Some expenses will be right away, some will be monthly, and some will be occasional, such as new walking shoes.

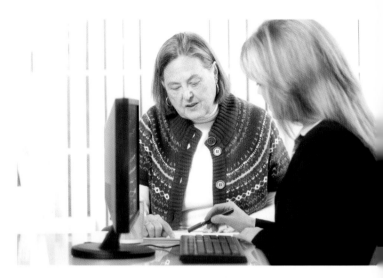

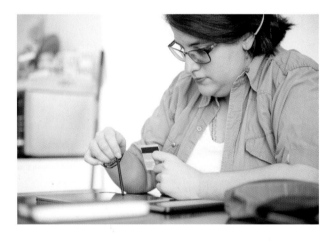

3 **Get help with your tax form if you need it.** Call community and family resource centers for free income tax advice and help. If you are low income and have not filled out a tax form for many years, the advisor will help you with the best options.

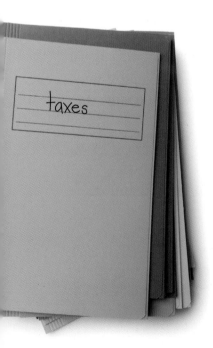

2 **Fill out your tax form each year.** You may not know about all the government cash-back benefits you could be eligible for. If you do not fill out your income tax form, you will not get the benefits. There are benefits for those who are not working, working but with a low income, seniors, those with disabilities and parents and their children.

4 **Get serious about budgeting.** This may help you deal with the new costs of diabetes, or with any related loss of income. A budget is your monthly or yearly list of income and expenses. Doing a budget can help you plan so you will spend less than you earn. Then you will have money left over for emergencies or planned special purchases.

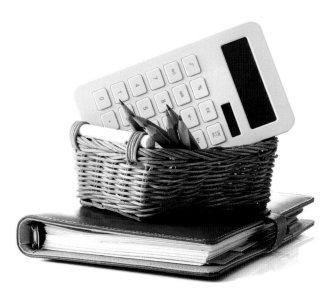

7 **Automatic bank transfer.** Have $20 taken off every paycheck and transferred into a savings account, and you will have $520 at the end of the year.

8 **Transportation.** Some cities have free bus passes or reduced taxi fares if you are low income, elderly or have a disability.

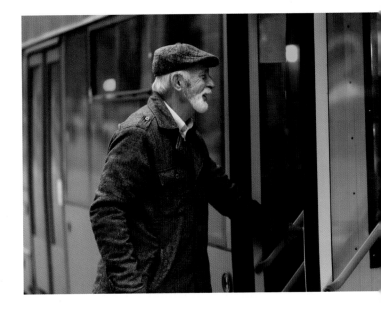

5 **Track spending for one month.** Write down every single cent you spent — every day for a month. Now you can make the first important choice for yourself: where you can cut back on your spending.

6 **A few ideas to save money.** Homemade meals are half the cost of restaurant meals. Think about buying fewer lottery tickets, less VLT time, fewer drinks from coffee shops and less impulse spending. Shop around for the pharmacy with the lowest pharmacy fees.

If you buy a coffee five days per week, bringing it from home could save you about $40 per month. That would be $480 in a year!

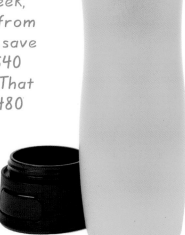

9 **Drug plans.** Ask for a list of medications covered by your drug plan. Veterans and Indigenous Americans or Canadians may be covered under a special drug plan. It may be easiest to have your health insurance fee as a monthly payment.

10 **Generic drugs.** They are identical to brand name drugs. If your drug plan does not pay for your diabetes medications, it might pay for the generic drugs or alternative drugs. If you are unable to pay for insulin, ask your doctor about financial aid for diabetes medications and supplies.

Having a Baby

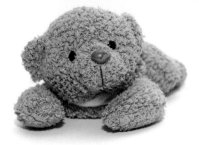

Plan before you get pregnant

1 **Improve your blood sugar.** Be more active and eat well. It can take three months to see an improvement in your blood sugar. This can be best assessed by your A1C level. Start your prenatal supplement now to build up your folic acid and iron levels.

2 **Drugs and alcohol.** If you smoke, drink alcohol or use cannabis or street drugs, talk to an addiction counselor about getting support to quit. Drugs and alcohol go directly to your baby. There is no safe amount.

3 **Tell your doctor about all your medications.** Medications include herbal supplements, over-the-counter and online medications. Some medications can harm a baby. Your doctor may discontinue some diabetes pills or replace them with insulin before you get pregnant.

Now you are pregnant

4 **A gradual weight gain is best.** Being pregnant does not mean eating as much as you want. Keep your portions controlled. The amount of weight you gain depends on your weight just before you got pregnant. Talk to your doctor about the right weight gain for you.

5 **Your baby needs healthy foods to grow.** Eat a wide variety of foods to keep your body healthy too. Meats and plant-based proteins give you iron; grains and starches give you energy and fiber; vegetables and fruits give you vitamins, while milk and milk products give you calcium and vitamin D. Continue with your prenatal vitamin.

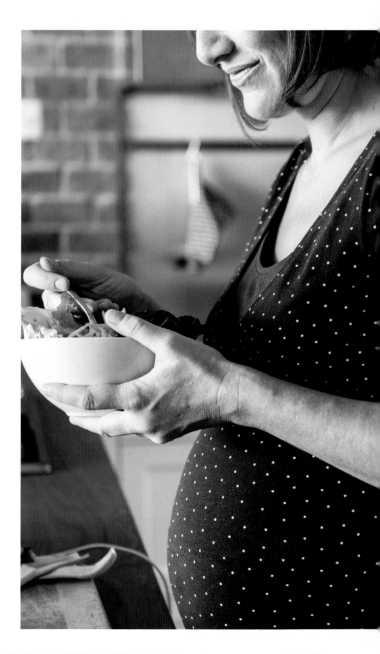

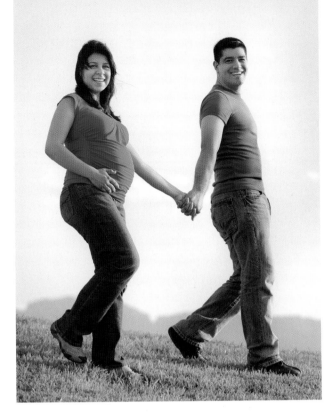

After your baby is born

9 **The benefits of breastfeeding.** Breastfeeding is recommended for you, even if you take insulin or diabetes pills. Your doctor may need to stop your meds or reduce your dose to prevent low blood sugar episodes. Here are some of the benefits:

- breastfeeding reduces your baby's future risk of type 2 diabetes
- it lowers your risk of breast cancer and heart disease
- women who have gestational diabetes get a special benefit — breastfeeding reduces their risk of going on to develop type 2 diabetes

Ask about having skin-to-skin time with your baby right after birth. This is known to help get breastfeeding started.

6 **Walk every day and do other exercise.** This helps prevent mom from gaining too much weight and reduces the risk of the baby getting too large. It also helps insulin work better to control blood sugar. Keep active unless your doctor recommends otherwise.

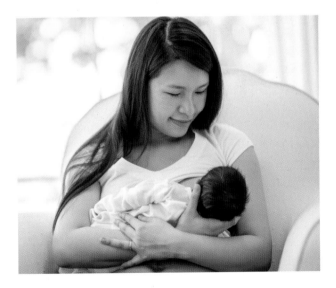

7 **Blood sugar tests are important.** The target ranges for blood sugar are different in pregnancy. Your doctor or diabetes educator may recommend you check your blood sugar at home more than usual, especially if you take insulin. You may need to come into the lab for more regular tests, especially in the third trimester when blood sugar goes the highest.

8 **Appointments.** See your doctor or midwife regularly. Have a diabetes eye exam in your first trimester, since pregnancy can increase the chance of damage to the back of your eyes.

10 **Birth control.** If you plan to have another baby, it is important to give your body a rest — plan for two years between births. This gives you time to return to your pre-pregnancy weight. Talk to your nurse or doctor about birth control options.

Tips to Prevent Type 2 Diabetes in Kids

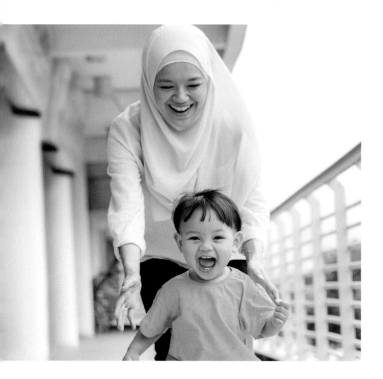

1 **Give your children the gift of health.** For children to feel safe and secure, you need to be available for them. So, turn off your phone at certain times and give them your full attention. This builds trust and it becomes easier for them to follow healthy rules.

2 **Early on, encourage active play.** Walk with them in strollers, visit playgrounds with climbing structures, and enjoy all-season, low-cost family outdoor activities, even walking to school. As they get older, encourage team sports. Some children may benefit from home exercise using a treadmill.

3 **Serve healthy foods at home.** Vegetables and fruit are important for the whole family. But children also need to learn that all foods can be chosen as part of a healthy diet in the right portions.

4 **Do not buy sweet drinks on a regular basis.** Drink water yourself, and offer water to your children. If you establish good habits at home when they are young, this will affect the choices they make as they grow up.

5 **Teach your children to cook.** This is an important life skill. Start with simple recipes. By the time they are teenagers, they can make dinner — hopefully!

Try making homemade pizza — see recipe on page 95.

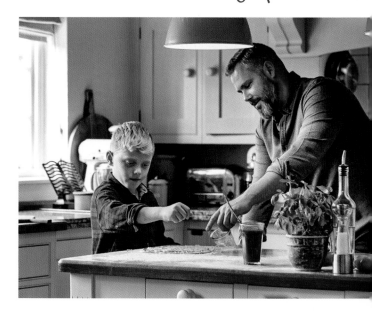

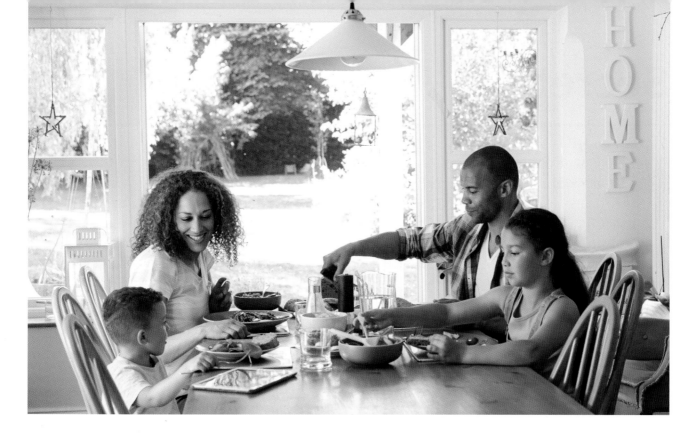

6 **Eat your meals together as a family.** Turn off all electronics. Research shows that when you eat together as a family, your children are not such picky eaters and are less likely to put on excess weight. When we eat together at home, we listen to each other's stories and talk about news of the day.

7 **Serve meals and snacks at regular times.** This helps reduce hunger. When children know their next meal or snack will be ready at the usual time, they learn to wait and not eat on impulse.

8 **Have a healthy attitude about weight no matter what you weigh.** When you talk about dieting or your own weight, you are heard as negative and being hard on yourself. Instead, talk about the good changes you are making and the importance of healthy foods and daily exercise. This will set a good example for your children.

9 **Do not smoke or vape around your children.** The same applies if you drink alcohol or smoke marijuana. You do not want your children to pick up these habits from you. Be the best role model you can.

10 **Limit screen time and cellphone time.** Seriously consider no television or tablet in your child's bedroom. Children need to read. Have many books at their reading level to encourage thinking and learning. Children need to learn to fall asleep without screens. Lengthy, uninterrupted sleep is critical to healthy brain growth and physical body development in children.

Secrets of Aging Well

1 **You may need less medication.** Many elderly people take more medications than they need, which may do more harm than good. As we age, our liver and kidneys do not clear out medications as well. This includes diabetes medication and insulin, which can build up in the blood and cause a low blood sugar episode.

2 **Prevent or reduce low blood sugar episodes.** If you have them often, your doctor may reduce or even stop your insulin or diabetes medication. The doctor may suggest new diabetes medications such as a GLP-1 or SGLT2, which cause fewer lows and have been proven to reduce heart attacks and strokes; see page 22–23. The doctor may also say that to reduce the risk of a low, it is safer to have a slightly higher blood sugar level after meals (up to 220 mg/dL USA or 12 mmol/L CAN).

3 **Treat low blood sugar episodes.** If you take insulin or diabetes pills that can cause a low blood sugar, keep glucose tablets in your pocket, on a bedside table, beside your favorite chair and in your car. Use a blood glucose meter to check your level before and after a low blood sugar episode.

4 **Rely on lists and other reminders.** Use a pill holder or pill blister pack from your pharmacist, to be sure you take your medications in the right order and at the right time. Write appointments on a calendar.

5 **Eat regular meals and drink water.** Good nutrition is important to fight a flu or cold, and it gives you the energy to do everyday activities. Drink water so you are less likely to get dehydrated or to get a urinary tract infection. If your appetite is poor, please read How to Gain Weight if You are Underweight, page 36–37.

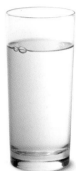

6 **Stay active.** Go for short walks with family or friends. Walking poles, a walking stick or a walker are great supports to keep you walking safely. Looking after your pet can also keep you active and provide company at the same time.

7 **Stay social.** Join a 55 Plus community group where you can play cards or do other activities and visit with other people your age. Attending church is meaningful, plus it is structured time to socialize and volunteer for church activities.

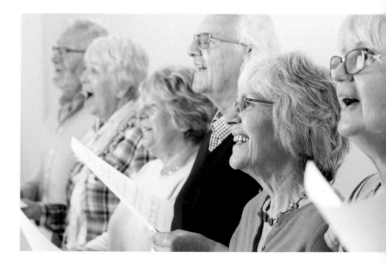

8 **If you live alone, wear an emergency medical alert system device at all times.** Should you fall at home and cannot get up to phone for help, push the alert button. Ask about devices that can tell if you have fallen and automatically alert the company, especially if you become unconscious.

10 **End of life planning.** This is something you probably think about. Be sure you have a legal and current will, and power of attorney. Talk to family members and your doctor about your wishes for a dignified passing. If you become very ill and cannot make your own decisions, it is less stressful for family if they know your wishes.

9 **Keep your routine.** As we get older, routines at a slower pace bring comfort. We appreciate regular meals and snacks and our favorite television shows. We anticipate at-home visits and outings with family and friends.

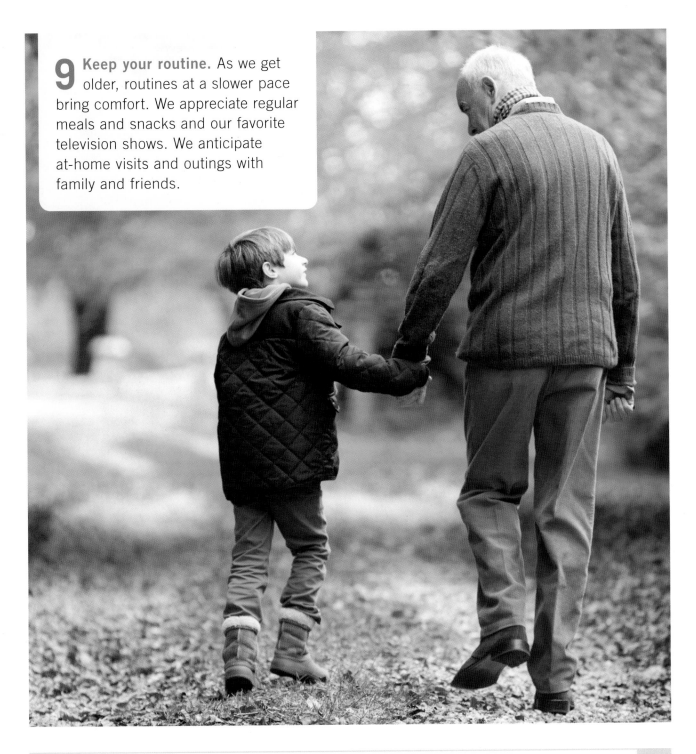

Being a Caregiver

1 **Someone who has had diabetes for many years may need a caregiver.** High blood sugar over many years damages the body and increases the risk for dementia, loss of hearing, reduced vision or blindness, a foot amputation, or kidney failure requiring home or clinic dialysis. As we live longer, we have an increased chance of having health issues where we will need help in day-to-day living.

2 **Who is a caregiver?** More of us will become a caregiver to someone else in our home, or family or friend's home. You may be a caregiver for a person with diabetes *and* have diabetes yourself. Sometimes it can be difficult work and sometimes it can be rewarding.

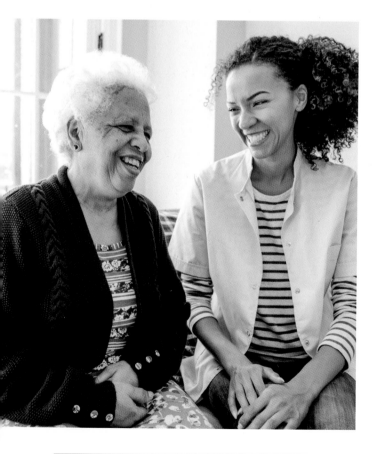

3 **As a caregiver, ask for help.** An occupational therapist or homecare nurse can come into your home to teach you new ways to give care, like how to bandage properly or how to operate a home dialysis machine.

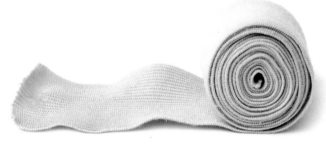

4 **Find community volunteers to help.** Community organizations will help you find volunteers to drive you to appointments, pick up groceries or cook for you, or stay in the home and provide short-term care while you do errands.

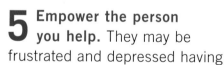

5 **Empower the person you help.** They may be frustrated and depressed having to depend on someone else to look after their daily needs. Install extra handrails in showers, and ramps to allow people in wheelchairs to be as independent as possible. There are many affordable devices to assist those who are losing their hearing or vision.

6 **Being a 24/7 caregiver can be difficult.** You may feel grief, anger and guilt. These are natural reactions to feeling overwhelmed. Being a caregiver for a family member can seem like never-ending, boring and sometimes unpleasant work. Take time for yourself to find a quiet place to relax and remember you both love each other and let the stressful moments pass.

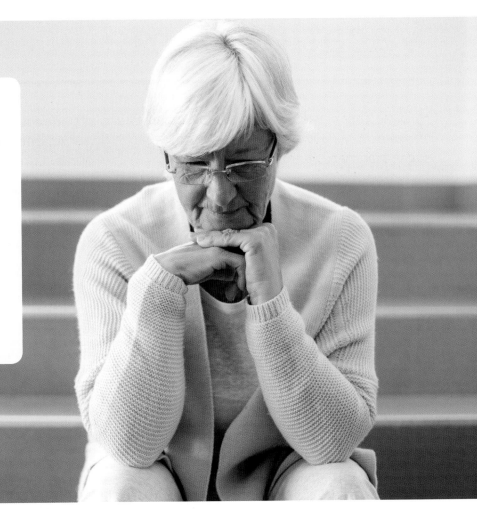

7 **Affection calms.** The person you are caring for will respond better through gentle touch and affection. When someone is not well, they need more time to think about what they want to say. So give space and time for talk to happen.

8 **Look after yourself.** Get outdoors for a short walk most days. If you cannot get a good night's sleep, could you sleep in a separate room? Eat healthy meals and drink plenty of water. Find time to watch your favorite television shows, to read, knit, or take a nap, and just do what you love to do. Be proud of the important caregiving that you are doing.

9 **Respite care.** Options include day programs or an overnight stay at a long-term care facility, supported in-part or fully by the government. Assessment by a nurse will be necessary prior to government respite care. Respite care gives you time off from being a caregiver. This makes it easier for you to continue to care for the person with diabetes in their home.

10 **Prepare for emergencies.** Write down on a sheet of paper their name and medical number, brief medical history, medications and allergies, their doctor's name and closest emergency contact. Put this on the front of the fridge for paramedics or take it with you to the hospital or clinic.

Vacation Time

1 **Have fun!** A vacation is often just what we need as a mental health break. Extra planning is important for a person with type 2 diabetes.

2 **Medical insurance.** If you get sick or need to be hospitalized in a foreign country, the costs without insurance can put your family in serious debt. Disclose all conditions and medications at the time you fill out the travel health insurance form.

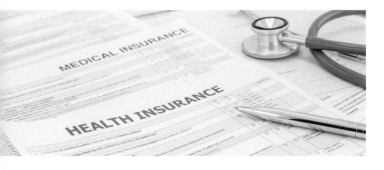

3 **Will and power of attorney.** Let your family know your health care wishes should you become too ill to make your own decisions while you are away from home.

4 **Carry diabetes identification.** Wear a medical alert bracelet. Set up the medical alert app on your smart phone for emergency responders to access. Or have a card in your wallet with your diabetes details.

5 **Reduce restaurant eating.** Most motel and hotel rooms have mini fridges and sinks. Carry a few plastic plates, bowls, cups and utensils, and buy groceries along the way. Carry a cooler in your vehicle for a healthy roadside picnic. See more information on page 62.

6 **Keep moving during long flights or road trips.** This helps blood circulation and reduces the risk of a blood clot. On a long flight, choose an aisle seat to get up and stretch your legs. On road trips, stop every hour or two for a short, brisk walk. Once you get to your vacation destination, continue with your daily walks.

7 **Carry-on bag with medications.** Place all medications, insulin, blood checking supplies and glucose tablets in one Ziploc bag. Insulin should go in an insulated container so it does not get too hot or too cold. Your medications must be in their original containers when going through customs. Include extra medications in case your trip is delayed. Include emergency medications such as anti-diarrheal.

8 **Important papers to include in your Ziploc bag.** Ask for a letter from your doctor explaining that you have type 2 diabetes and the medications you are carrying. Also include a copy of your sick day plan (please see page 32).

9 **Adjust medications and insulin so you transition gradually when flying through time zones.** Before you leave on an international trip, talk to your health care provider to develop a medication schedule. If you fly across time zones regularly, it is helpful to have an insulin pump or long or ultra-long insulin as your background insulin, combined with a rapid insulin that is taken just before you eat. Continuous glucose monitoring is very helpful too. Even with the best planning there are blood sugar ups and downs.

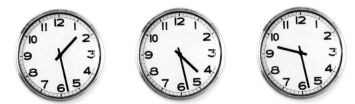

10 **Jet lag.** If possible, allow an extra day at the beginning and end of your vacation to rest and get used to the new time zone. Jet lag changes your sleep rhythms and can disrupt your medication schedule.

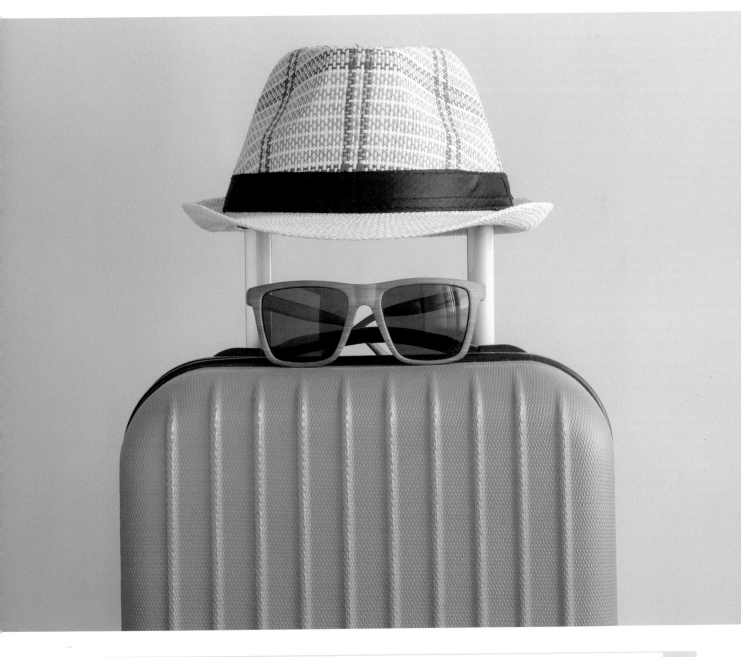

Promising New Research

1 **Creating healthier spaces to live.** City planners are building green spaces, walking paths, cycling lanes and venues for accessible active sports. More is needed to help us live healthier.

2 **Protect and support children.** Research on Adverse Childhood Experiences (ACE's) shows that the more trauma a child experiences, the more likely that they will develop physical and mental health problems, including diabetes. In fact, research is confirming that ACE's have a stronger link to diabetes than genetics do. A healthy child becomes a healthy adult.

3 **Diabetes Prevention Program studies.** Research has shown that people with prediabetes who received initial and ongoing support from medical workers, educators and coaches to make healthy changes lowered their risk of developing type 2 diabetes by 58%. Good support allows for healthy living and less diabetes.

4 **Diabetes Prevention Program study of metformin.** Researchers are examining whether early metformin use reduces the long-term risk for diabetes, and for heart disease and cancer. In the first five-year phase of the study, the metformin group were 31% less likely to develop type 2 diabetes. Metformin is an older drug but a good one.

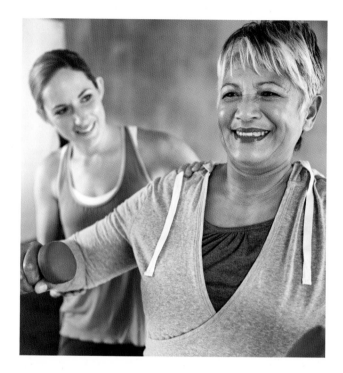

5 **New UK study links weight loss to possible remission of diabetes.** The two-year study, called DiRECT, involved participants with type 2 diabetes who were not on insulin. Each person started with a body mass index (BMI) of between 27 and 45. They got intensive medical support and coaching. For the first three months, their diabetes and blood pressure meds were stopped. Their food was replaced with nutrient-supplemented shakes (about 850 calories a day). A 30-lb (15 kg) weight loss was common after the three months. Then they transitioned back to a diet of 2,000 calories or less and participated in an active exercise program. For about one third of participants, this helped maintain their weight loss and their diabetes went into remission to the end of the two-year study. The study is continuing and this research will assess the long-term risks and benefits.

6 **Improved diabetes medications.** Today there are seven main groups of diabetes medications compared to only two groups 30 years ago. Drug companies have combined two different diabetes medications into one convenient pill and have produced medications that can be taken just once a week. Many medications have been developed that lower blood sugar and weight, and also reduce the risk of heart failure, heart attack and stroke. Ask your doctor about the new and latest medications.

· ·

7 **New insulins.** Research is aimed at developing ultra-rapid and ultra-long insulins. Afrezza (approved in the USA) is a new device where ultra-rapid insulin is inhaled with a puffer rather than injected. It can be an add-on to other medications, when sugar levels spike. Still in the early research stage are "smart insulins" that will turn on or off in response to blood sugar levels. If one type of insulin isn't working, ask your doctor about other types.

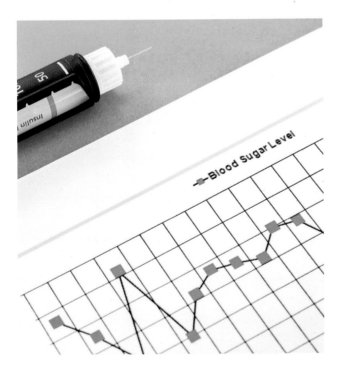

8 **No more finger pricking for blood sugars.** One method is a computerized sensor patch that is placed on the arm and transmits sugar levels to your phone or watch. Another type of sensor is implanted under the skin to read sugar levels for six months at a time. There are sensors that clip on the earlobe and read blood sugar through sound waves, heat and electromagnetics. In development is a smart contact lens that reads blood sugar levels in tears. In addition, tattoos made of glucose-responsive inks will change color with sugar levels.

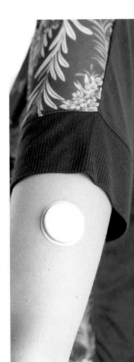

· ·

9 **The artificial pancreas device.** One part continuously reads blood sugar levels and another part delivers the right amount of insulin (and sometimes other hormones like glucagon). Trial models are used by people with type 1 diabetes. They are being developed to be smaller and more accurate and may in the future be used by people with type 2 diabetes.

· ·

10 **Bariatric surgery to reduce the size of the stomach.** Bariatric surgery has become a more common and promising surgery. When performed by an experienced surgeon there are fewer risks, although you need lifelong follow-up after the surgery. It may be recommended as an option for someone with diabetes who has a body mass index (BMI) of over 35, who has been unable to lose weight with diet and exercise. After surgery, people are less hungry, eat much less, and so usually lose a lot of weight. The diabetes can even go into remission.

Ten Diabetes Quizzes

Test Your Knowledge!

Take your time to do the quizzes and read the answers through. After you've done the quiz, you can check the answers on the reverse page.

If you write your answers in your own notebook, you can try the quizzes again in a few months or a year, and you may have different answers. 10 out of 10 is the best score possible. 7 is a pretty awesome score too!

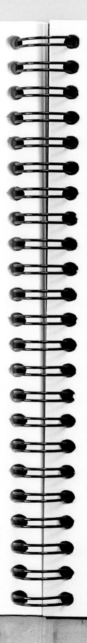

Diabetes Knowledge Quiz

QUESTION	TRUE	FALSE
1. If you have prediabetes you should start making lifestyle changes right away.	◯	◯
2. Thin people do not get type 2 diabetes.	◯	◯
3. A good night's sleep may help lower your morning fasting blood sugar.	◯	◯
4. Oxytocin and endorphins are two types of hormones that make your blood sugar go up.	◯	◯
5. As long as I feel well, I don't have to check my blood sugar at home or go for an A1C test.	◯	◯
6. Insulin is the only diabetes medication given by injection.	◯	◯
7. Unsweetened apple juice has more sugar than regular Coke or Pepsi.	◯	◯
8. High blood sugar can cause infection in the gums.	◯	◯
9. A diabetes eye check-up is recommended once every three years.	◯	◯
10. With proper foot care, most diabetes foot ulcers and amputations can be prevented.	◯	◯

How did you do? Add up all of your right answers, found on page 170.
Your Score: ____ out of 10.

Diabetes Knowledge Answers

1 **True.** If changes are made at the prediabetes stage, there is a very good chance that type 2 diabetes can be prevented. Go for regular check-ups; this includes a blood sugar test once a year. Your doctor may prescribe a diabetes pill.

2 **False.** For thin people, type 2 diabetes is more likely when they get older; if they have a strong family history of diabetes; if they smoke; or if they have high blood pressure or high triglycerides.

3 **True.** When you are sound asleep your body releases less cortisol, which results in a decrease of blood sugar. A good night's sleep helps your insulin work better, so your morning fasting blood sugar will be lower.

4 **False.** Oxytocin and endorphins help you relax and feel good, which decreases blood sugar. Oxytocin is released when you cuddle or feel loved, and endorphins when you exercise.

5 **False.** Don't assume that because you feel fine your blood sugar is fine. Your blood sugar can gradually rise, your body can adapt, and you may not notice the change. Blood sugar checks are very important.

6 **False.** Diabetes medications given by injection include brand names such as Byetta, Bydureon, Ozempic, Trulicity and Victoza. These newer drugs do not cause weight gain or low blood sugar episodes.

7 **True.** One cup (250 mL) of unsweetened apple juice has 7½ teaspoons of sugar (30 grams of carbohydrate). One cup (250 mL) of regular Coke or Pepsi has 6½ teaspoons of sugar (26 grams of carbohydrate).

8 **True.** To slow down or stop gum disease, you need good blood sugar control. Floss every day, and brush your teeth with a soft toothbrush.

9 **False.** Make an appointment with an optometrist soon after diagnosis of diabetes, and then every year, or as recommended. Regular eye exams catch problems early so they can be treated.

10 **True.** Have your nurse or doctor screen your feet for nerve damage (neuropathy). Check your feet daily, apply cream, wear proper shoes and socks, and treat all sores and cuts right away.

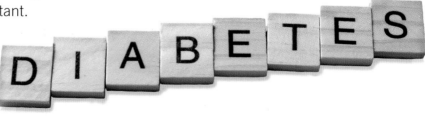

Your Diabetes Health Quiz

QUESTION	YES	NO
1. Every day, I take time to relax.	○	○
2. I eat quickly — I usually finish a meal in less than five minutes.	○	○
3. In the last year, I have gone on a strict diet.	○	○
4. Most days, I sit for more than eight hours. Sitting includes driving, watching TV or sitting at a desk.	○	○
5. Most nights I sleep about 7 hours.	○	○
6. Every day, I drink more than two cups of sugary drinks or unsweetened fruit juice.	○	○
7. Every week, I have seven or more alcoholic drinks.	○	○
8. Every day, I eat two or more different vegetables.	○	○
9. I smoke cigarettes or e-cigarettes.	○	○
10. Every day, I look at the tops and bottoms of my feet.	○	○

How did you do? Add up all of your right answers, found on page 172.
Your Score: ____ out of 10.

Your Diabetes Health Answers

1 **Yes.** Relaxation pays off. Research shows that people who live long and healthy lives have ways to relax every day.

2 **No.** Be mindful when you eat to prevent overeating. Slow down your eating; take smaller mouthfuls; put your utensils down between bites; and drink water with your meals.

3 **No.** Eat healthy. Strict diets cause fast and large weight loss. Research shows that without long-term lifestyle change, that once "off" the diet, almost all of these dieters regain that weight, and some gain even more than before their diet. However, if you answered "Yes," some new evidence shows that with intensive medical and lifestyle support, a short-term low-calorie diet can help maintain weight loss over a longer term (see page 166).

4 **No.** Move more. Too much sitting is associated with a rise in blood sugar, blood pressure and weight gain.

5 **Yes.** Seven hours of sleep is good for most people. When you do not get enough sleep, your appetite hormones get disrupted and you will feel hungrier and eat more during the day.

6 **No.** Limit sugary drinks and juice. These have a lot of calories and will contribute to weight gain.

7 **No.** Limit alcohol. Alcohol is addictive. The calories from alcohol can quickly add up to weight gain.

8 **Yes.** Say yes to vegetables. When you eat vegetables and fruits every day, you get more vitamins and antioxidants, which help keep your blood vessels healthy.

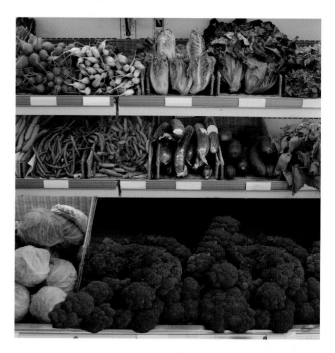

9 **No.** Seek help to quit or smoke less. People with diabetes who smoke are more likely to have a heart attack or stroke or develop nerve damage in their feet.

10 **Yes.** Care for your feet — it's worth it! Treat sores and cuts immediately. You want to prevent an infection that could lead to an ulcer or amputation.

Weight Loss Quiz

QUESTION	YES	NO
1. I eat take-out or in a restaurant twice a week or more.	○	○
2. I often shop for groceries when I am hungry.	○	○
3. During some holidays, I have gained five or more pounds.	○	○
4. I write in my notebook or app my weight loss progress.	○	○
5. When I feel stressed I eat more food, especially junk food.	○	○
6. I often skip meals.	○	○
7. Most days, I walk or do other exercise for 15 minutes or more.	○	○
8. After binge eating, it is best to get back to healthy eating for the next meal.	○	○
9. Right now, I am too busy to do anything about my weight or my weight gain.	○	○
10. I believe I can lose five or 10 pounds.	○	○

How did you do? Add up all of your right answers, found on page 174.
Your Score: ____ out of 10.

Weight Loss Answers

1 **No.** Eat at home more often. Restaurant portions are usually oversized, over-salted and fattening.

2 **No.** Plan grocery shopping. Make a list of healthy foods to buy, and shop when you are not hungry. People tend to buy more food when they are hungry.

3 **No.** Do not ignore holiday weight gain. Doctors say that if you quickly gain five or more pounds due to holiday overeating, you should treat it as a medical emergency. Do not delay, get back on track. The good news is — it is easier to lose extra weight in the first month after you have gained it.

4 **Yes.** Keep track to keep motivated. Keep daily notes on the number of steps you take, how many hours you sleep, how many hours you sit, your screen time, your blood pressure, your blood sugar, or your weight or your waist measurement.

5 **No.** Explore healthy new ways to relax and manage stress. Get dressed for the weather and go outside, play music or a game on your phone, read, enjoy a cup of tea, find quiet time alone, or nap for 15 minutes.

6 **No.** Eat at regular times. During the day, have a meal or snack every three hours so you will be less likely to overeat at the next meal or snack.

7 **Yes.** Be active. Start with a 10- or 15-minute walk today. Gradually do more when you are ready. If you can build up to a 30-minute walk every day, this is the best medicine to keep you healthy.

8 **Yes.** Set yourself up for success. Eat smaller portions during the day and drink lots of water.

9 **No.** Being "too busy" may be an excuse. If you are not eating and exercising properly you will gain weight. Be positive and tell yourself you are never too busy to keep yourself healthy.

10 **Yes.** Believe in yourself. Seek out good support to eat well and be active. This might be a dietitian or nurse, a doctor, a trainer at a gym, a friend, or your partner who may join you in losing weight.

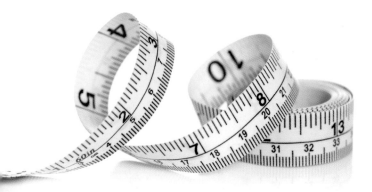

How You Think Quiz

QUESTION	YES	NO
1. I see things as all or nothing. I overate last night — I'm such a failure.	○	○
2. I try to look for the positive in a situation. Rather than focus on my high blood sugars, I look at the good numbers to understand what I did well.	○	○
3. People tell me I jump to conclusions or overthink things. The doctor probably thinks I am a loser.	○	○
4. I try to change everything all at once.	○	○
5. I believe I should be rewarded with my favorite foods regularly.	○	○
6. I feel that no matter what I do I will get diabetes complications, so what is the use of even trying.	○	○
7. Managing my diabetes takes more than medications.	○	○
8. I am too shy to say no when people offer me another helping.	○	○
9. I like to get my money's worth for my meal deal.	○	○
10. I am too old to learn, and I believe in the saying, "You cannot teach an old dog new tricks."	○	○

How did you do? Add up all of your right answers, found on page 176.
Your Score: ___ out of 10.

How You Think Answers

1 **No.** Negative self-talk offers you no choices. Rarely are things all bad or all good. Ask yourself, "Is there a better way to look at this situation?"

2 **Yes.** Think about what you do well. Positive thinking releases relaxing hormones, which improve blood sugar levels. A small shift in how you think can motivate you to make a positive health change.

3 **No.** Look at the situation in a new way. We may overthink when we try to guess what others are thinking. Both words and silences are often misunderstood. It's hard to really know the intention of another person. Ask people what they meant by what they said.

4 **No.** Write down small goals that are realistic. Over the next week I will go for a 15-minute walk three times. Reaching goals helps you feel good about yourself.

5 **No.** Your best reward is your good health from exercise and healthy eating. Be aware, food advertisements constantly tell us that we deserve a break and need food rewards. Food ads encourage overeating.

6 **No.** Changes will make a difference. A small daily change can improve your A1C level to reduce the risk of eye, kidney and nerve damage. Small daily actions include: move about more, smoke less, check your feet, and take your diabetes or blood pressure medication. You can do it!

7 **Yes.** Medications alone are not enough. Medications treat the symptoms of diabetes but daily exercise and eating well will slow the progression of diabetes and the development of complications.

8 **No.** Practice being assertive. Politely say "no thanks." With practice it gets easier. Your friends begin to understand that you are serious about your changes.

9 **No.** The best deal when you have diabetes is a small meal that is not fried. The larger the meal, the higher your blood sugar will go. Think about eating out less.

10 **No.** We can always learn, no matter what our age. Learning happens when we socialize with friends, play games, do hobbies, volunteer, join community groups or attend local cultural events. Learning keeps our brains and bodies alert.

Stress Management Quiz

QUESTION	YES	NO
1. I worry about my health and family matters, or about school or work, or about money.	◯	◯
2. I have someone I can talk to about my personal feelings.	◯	◯
3. Life is so busy I have no time to relax.	◯	◯
4. High blood pressure is a sign of stress.	◯	◯
5. I understand that mental health and physical health are connected.	◯	◯
6. "Winter blues" are more common in people who live in northern climates.	◯	◯
7. Most mornings when I wake up, I feel rested.	◯	◯
8. I feel overwhelmed by the tasks at home or work.	◯	◯
9. I believe laughter is good medicine.	◯	◯
10. I feel my life has no meaning and no purpose.	◯	◯

How did you do? Add up all of your right answers, found on page 178.
Your Score: ____ out of 10.

Stress Management Answers

1 **No.** Worry does not change things. Changes need action. Let people know you are worried about them. If school or work is overwhelming, have conversations with people who can help you. If you have debt and cannot manage payments, most community resource centers offer free counseling to help with budgeting.

2 **Yes.** Seek support. Talk with your partner, call a friend or family member, reach out for support to your doctor or health care provider, a spiritual advisor or a diabetes online support group.

3 **No.** Build relaxation into your life. People who live long and healthy lives find positive ways to relax every day. Take a few minutes to close your eyes and focus on relaxing.

4 **Yes.** Moderate to high stress can cause high blood pressure. Talk with your doctor about what brings stress into your life.

5 **Yes.** Seek professional help when you need it. It helps to talk to someone about your personal issues. You will get new ideas and find solutions, even small ones.

6 **Yes.** "Winter blues" are more common in northern climates. Special fluorescent lights that act like sunlight can help. A walk outdoors, summer or winter, especially in sunlight, is like a boost of energy.

7 **Yes.** A good night's sleep produces relaxing hormones. Remember to darken your room and turn off all electronics about half an hour before bedtime. A walk during the day or early evening helps tire you and prepare you for sleep.

8 **No.** Organize your time with a to-do list. Sort your list into essential jobs. Do one task at a time. Check off tasks as you get them done — yes, that feels good!

9 **Yes.** Humor and laughter balance life. Laughter releases feel-good hormones. A sense of humor helps us see that some things are not such big issues.

10 **No.** It is common to feel a sense of hopelessness with the diagnosis of type 2 diabetes. It can be difficult to see how the changes will improve your future. Changes are going to take your time and your commitment. You will learn to manage diabetes and then you can share your personal experience and information with others. You are an important person to many people who need you to be healthy.

How to Improve Sex Quiz

QUESTION	YES	NO
1. I feel comfortable talking to my doctor about issues with my sex life.	○	○
2. I believe that eating well and regular exercise can improve the sexual health of a person with diabetes.	○	○
3. I feel anxious that I may not perform well or satisfy my partner or myself.	○	○
4. My sex routine is always the same.	○	○
5. I like to set the mood.	○	○
6. Erectile dysfunction can be handled best if both partners look for solutions together.	○	○
7. If a man with diabetes has problems achieving a firm erection, Viagra can often help.	○	○
8. I believe it is safe to buy sexual aids online.	○	○
9. Could these medications strengthen a man's erection: antihistamines, antidepressants, tranquilizers or ulcer drugs?	○	○
10. I tell my partner what makes me feel happy in and out of the bedroom.	○	○

How did you do? Add up all of your right answers, found on page 180.
Your Score: ____ out of 10.

How to Improve Sex Answers

1 **Yes.** Talk to your doctor or diabetes educator. By talking, you give the doctor permission to give you information without judging you.

2 **Yes.** There are thousands of touch-sensitive pleasure nerves on our skin. Healthy foods keep these nerves firing. Regular exercise increases blood flow, oxygen and nitric oxide to these nerves and surrounding blood vessels.

3 **No.** Reduce anxiety. Talk about what you like, and listen to your partner. Talk about your past fun sexual times together.

4 **No.** Change things up. Try a new place or a new position, or a vibrator with a lubricant.

5 **Yes.** Build the mood. Earlier in the day, text your intentions and ask if your partner agrees. Share a meal together. Give your partner a loving neck rub.

6 **Yes.** Explore ways together to satisfy each other. Yes, respectful partners are essential to a healthy sexual relationship. When a couple feel sexually content, these feelings can extend to improve everything in their relationship.

7 **Yes.** Viagra-like medications, called PDE5's, can often help with firmness. They are a good solution for many men, including those with diabetes. Your doctor may recommend other types of erectile medications. Caution: Don't order pills or herbal aphrodisiacs online without checking with your doctor. They are mostly unregulated and may be unsafe.

8 **No.** Buy sexual aids only from online stores with a 1-800 phone support line such as Amazon. This precaution is needed to avoid unwanted ads and spam for offending pornographic material. Keep your computer safe for all family members to use.

9 **No.** These meds have the possible side effect to weaken a man's erection. The good news is a man can often offset this side effect by planning his sexual activities for a time when his medication is not peaking. The doctor may also suggest alternative medications.

10 **Yes.** Consider your own needs, even if they're different from your partner's needs. Often, it's women who hesitate to do this. But it's important to speak up. Make sure you're comfortable with new positions. Some lubricants may not be suitable for you. Let your partner know what works, what doesn't, and what you prefer.

Get Active Quiz

QUESTION	TRUE	FALSE
1. Jogging is the best exercise for a person with type 2 diabetes who is overweight.	◯	◯
2. High-repetition strength training or resistance-band exercises help lower blood sugar over the long term.	◯	◯
3. Exercise helps improve how well insulin works.	◯	◯
4. When I am more active, I need to eat extra protein to build muscle.	◯	◯
5. I should not walk when I have pain in both my calves.	◯	◯
6. Walking reduces constipation.	◯	◯
7. Walking poles will not help me walk longer.	◯	◯
8. In hot weather, it is best to go barefoot or wear sandals, so my feet do not overheat.	◯	◯
9. When I go for a walk, I should carry a chocolate bar to treat a low blood sugar episode.	◯	◯
10. Adults who walk or do daily exercise get many health benefits.	◯	◯

How did you do? Add up all of your right answers, found on page 182.
Your Score: ____ out of 10.

Get Active Answers

1 False. Jogging can hurt the bottom of your feet, your leg joints and even the back of your eyes (a concern for those with diabetes retinopathy). Jogging is an intense exercise that causes fast blood sugar highs and lows, which can make you hungry and overeat.

2 True. Over the long term, strength training is good for people with diabetes; it helps insulin work better, and lower blood sugar is the result. However, if you check your blood sugar right after strength training, it may read higher than expected. This is because the hormones adrenalin and cortisol are released, which temporarily raises blood sugar.

3 True. Insulin continues to work better for 12 to 24 hours after exercise. Once you become more active, you can usually cut back on your insulin.

4 False. Extra protein adds extra calories. Stick with a healthy balanced diet and muscles will build strength naturally with exercise.

5 False. Pain in both your calves may be due to poor blood circulation, which means less oxygen to the muscles and veins in your legs. For this, doctors recommend that you walk a few minutes, then stop; then "walk and stop" again. If the pain worsens or is just in one leg always seek your doctor's advice.

6 True. Walking is the best exercise to keep your bowels moving. Drinking water and eating high fiber foods also helps.

7 False. Walking poles are the best! Walking poles take pressure off sore joints. This means less pain and you can walk more. When people see you walking with your poles they know that you care about your safety and good health.

8 False. Heat dries the skin on your feet and heels. This can cause cracks that can become infected. A stubbed toe can also lead to an injury, which may take longer to heal. Properly fitted shoes are always the right thing to wear all year.

9 False. You need quick sugar to treat a low blood sugar episode. Carry glucose tablets in your pocket. A chocolate bar has sugar *and* fat. Fat slows the sugar from entering your bloodstream.

10 True. Exercise improves circulation, breathing and mobility. It boosts immunity, helps insulin work better, and can help prevent weight gain. Research is continuing to prove that exercise has so many benefits, even reducing dementia — have a healthy mind for longer.

Quit Smoking Quiz

QUESTION	TRUE	FALSE
1. It is easy for people who are light smokers to quit.	○	○
2. It is my choice to smoke, this does not affect others in my life.	○	○
3. Most people quit more than once before they become a non-smoker for good.	○	○
4. The only way to quit smoking is "cold turkey."	○	○
5. Nicotine replacement therapy, such as the nicotine patch, has been proven to help people quit.	○	○
6. A good way to quit smoking cigarettes is to switch to e-cigarettes (vaping or juuling).	○	○
7. I need a plan for how I will manage after I quit.	○	○
8. Most people who quit smoking gain some weight.	○	○
9. Smoking increases the risk for diabetes complications.	○	○
10. After I quit, my blood pressure will go down.	○	○

How did you do? Add up all of your right answers, found on page 184.
Your Score: ____ out of 10.

Quit Smoking Answers

1 False. Smoking is an addiction. All smokers have different mental health strengths, social lives, home situations and genetic factors that all play a part in the addiction. Quitting the smoking addiction takes as much commitment from light smokers as heavy smokers.

2 False. Smoking affects family and friends who worry about your health. The cost of cigarettes affects family income. And second-hand smoke is unpleasant and unhealthy for all who breathe it in.

3 True. No matter how many cigarettes a person smokes, there will usually be many tries before they become a non-smoker.

4 False. Studies show that people have better success if they cut back slowly over several weeks and use nicotine replacement therapy (NRT).

5 True. People are even more successful at quitting when they connect with a smoking cessation counselor.

6 False. E-cigarettes do not list the amount of nicotine, so they are not a reliable nicotine replacement product.

7 True. Before quit day, make a plan for healthy food and drinks; a plan for a daily exercise routine; and a plan to keep your hands busy. Having a plan will increase your chances of success.

8 True. An average weight gain is 5 to 10 lbs (2 to $4\frac{1}{2}$ kg). However, with your plan for exercise and healthy foods, weight gain can be prevented. A really great benefit of exercise is that it increases your metabolism.

9 True. Nicotine from smoking narrows and damages blood vessels and nerves and decreases the flow of oxygen to your muscles. All this damage to the body leads to diabetes complications, which include a higher risk for heart attack, stroke, foot amputation, dialysis, loss of vision and, for men, erectile dysfunction.

10 True. It is proven that within half an hour of quitting, your blood pressure can improve. You will breathe more easily and feel like a much healthier person.

Diabetes Do's and Don'ts Quiz

QUESTION	DO	DON'T
1. Have several alcoholic drinks in the evening to help reduce swelling in your legs.	○	○
2. Apply moisturizer cream once a day to the tops of your feet, between your toes, and on your heels.	○	○
3. If you have a low blood sugar episode while driving, take 15 grams of glucose tablets and continue driving.	○	○
4. If you are pregnant, aim for a 25 to 35 pound weight gain (11–16 kg).	○	○
5. Find the spot on your body where it is most comfortable to inject your insulin or diabetes medication, and continue to use this spot.	○	○
6. Cut your toenails straight across.	○	○
7. After a half-hour walk, have a sports drink to replenish your sugar and salt.	○	○
8. See a doctor if have muscle cramps, dark colored pee, are very thirsty and are feeling confused.	○	○
9. If you see one or two high blood sugar readings, change your dosage of insulin or diabetes pills right away.	○	○
10. Whole grain bread has a low glycemic index, so eat as much as you want.	○	○

How did you do? Add up all of your right answers, found on page 186.
Your Score: ____ out of 10.

Diabetes Do's and Don'ts Answers

1 **DON'T drink alcohol for this reason.** And don't drink it more than moderately at all. It actually causes your body to hold more water, which can increase swelling.

2 **DON'T put moisturizer between your toes.** Dry between the toes to avoid a fungal infection.

3 **DON'T continue to drive.** Pull over and stop as soon as you can. Treat your low blood sugar episode immediately with 15 grams of glucose tablets. If you do not have sugar with you, stay parked and phone for help. For safety, you should not drive for 40 minutes after a low. Recheck your blood sugar before driving again; it should read 90 mg/dL USA (5.0 mmol/L CAN) or higher.

4 **DO gain this amount of weight, unless your doctor recommends that you gain more or less.** Pregnancy is not a reason to be inactive and overeat. If you gain too much weight too quickly, you increase the chance of having a large baby. Larger babies are more difficult to deliver; they have more complications at birth; and they have a greater risk of developing diabetes later in life.

5 **DON'T inject in the same spot over and over.** This can cause a hard lump of fat to develop under the skin at the injection site. Insulin is then poorly absorbed at this site.

6 **DO trim your toenails straight across and file the sharp edges with a nail file.** Don't cut the nails too short.

7 **DON'T drink sports drinks.** These drinks are created for competitive athletes and marathon runners who sweat hard and lose important minerals in their sweat. Drinking water is all the fluid replacement you will need.

8 **DO seek help immediately.** Together these are signs of serious dehydration. This can happen if you are vomiting or have diarrhea. When you are dehydrated your blood sugar level will be high.

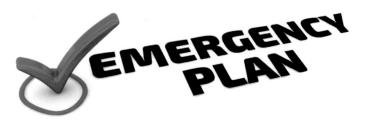

9 **DON'T change your medications based on just one or two results.** Make changes based on trends. A trend is a similar pattern over several days or a week.

10 **DON'T overeat whole grain bread.** Lower glycemic breads still increase blood sugar, it is just that the rise is slower than other carbohydrates. Enjoy a slice or two.

Diabetes After One Year Quiz

QUESTION	YES	NO
1. I spend a lot of time alone, and little time with friends, family or co-workers.	◯	◯
2. I walk or do other aerobic-type exercise for 25 or more minutes a day.	◯	◯
3. Every day, I drink four or more cups of water.	◯	◯
4. I eat breakfast every morning.	◯	◯
5. One day a week or more my meals are meatless.	◯	◯
6. I have home-cooked meals four or more times a week.	◯	◯
7. Every day I brush my teeth or dentures.	◯	◯
8. Once a day I check my feet to make sure there are no sores.	◯	◯
9. After I eat, I often feel guilty.	◯	◯
10. I see my doctor or diabetes educator for a diabetes check-up two or more times a year.	◯	◯

How did you do? Add up all of your right answers, found on page 188.
Your Score: ____ out of 10.

Diabetes After One Year Answers

1 **No.** Connecting with others can help us manage stress more easily. It feels good to have healthy, caring relationships with people we like. The body responds and releases oxytocin, an anti-stress hormone that improves blood sugar.

2 **Yes.** Exercise is crucial; 25 minutes is the minimum daily amount recommended for adults by the American Diabetes Association and Diabetes Canada. Exercise helps insulin work better and can help prevent weight gain.

3 **Yes.** Drink water. Water helps prevent dehydration. It helps reduce constipation. It helps reduce the risk of a urinary tract infection. And it helps you feel less hungry so you do not overeat.

4 **Yes.** Breakfast is the most important meal of the day. It is the "fuel that turns on your engine" to burn stored fat. Eat less food in the evening so you will be ready to eat in the morning.

5 **Yes.** Vegetable protein is easier on your kidneys. Beans and lentils are low in fat and high in fiber. Add dried beans, peas or lentils to soups and stews. Rinse canned kidney beans or lentils to reduce salt.

6 **Yes.** Eat more home-cooked meals. You control the portion sizes, the amount of added salt, fat and sugar; you will save money and feel healthier.

7 **Yes.** Look after your gums and teeth. Brush and floss every day. When your blood sugar is high, you are more likely to get a gum infection, so caring for your teeth is especially important.

8 **Yes.** Look after your feet. When you have type 2 diabetes, you may not feel a sore or cut on your foot. You want to treat your sores immediately to avoid an infection.

9 **No.** Guilt is an emotion focused on the past that you cannot change now. Instead, focus on the gains you have made. If you overeat at a meal, plan for the next day to return to your healthy way of eating and start with breakfast.

10 **Yes.** Regular doctor's appointments are important. People who have regular appointments get support for necessary changes and are better informed to manage their diabetes.

21 Doctor!

Index

THERE ARE THREE BOOKS IN OUR HEALTH & WELLNESS SERIES

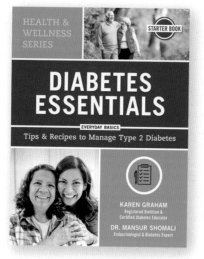

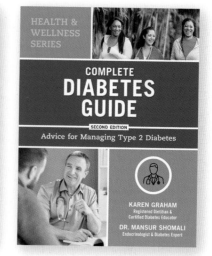

Did you just find out you have type 2 diabetes? *Diabetes Essentials* answers all your first questions.

Are you struggling with what meals to make? Turn to the *Diabetes Cookbook* for complete meal planning.

Do you need more information about diabetes? It's time to go to the *Complete Diabetes Guide.*

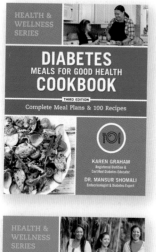

Features:

- Life-size photos of meals and snacks
- An "Eat This–Not That" section, comparing common foods and beverages to help you choose between them
- Weight loss guide, using daily meal plans from 1,200 to 2,200 calories
- Recipes and meals for type 1 or type 2 diabetes, listing carbohydrates and key nutrients

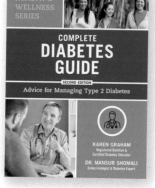

Features:

- Easy-to-understand information about diabetes
- Every diabetes topic covered, such as food choices, stress management and foot care
- Recommendations on how to prevent and reduce diabetes complications
- Reliable information on diabetes medications and technologies

AVAILABLE WHEREVER BOOKS ARE SOLD